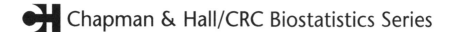
Chapman & Hall/CRC Biostatistics Series

Computational
Pharmacokinetics

Chapman & Hall/CRC Biostatistics Series

Editor-in-Chief

Shein-Chung Chow, Ph.D.
Professor
Department of Biostatistics and Bioinformatics
Duke University School of Medicine
Durham, North Carolina, U.S.A.

Series Editors

Byron Jones
Senior Director
Statistical Research and Consulting Centre
(IPC 193)
Pfizer Global Research and Development
Sandwich, Kent, UK

Jen-pei Liu
Professor
Division of Biometry
Department of Agronomy
National Taiwan University
Taipei, Taiwan

Karl E. Peace
Director, Karl E. Peace Center for Biostatistics
Professor of Biostatistics
Georgia Cancer Coalition Distinguished Cancer Scholar
Georgia Southern University, Statesboro, GA

CH Chapman & Hall/CRC Biostatistics Series

Published Titles

1. *Design and Analysis of Animal Studies in Pharmaceutical Development,* Shein-Chung Chow and Jen-pei Liu
2. *Basic Statistics and Pharmaceutical Statistical Applications,* James E. De Muth
3. *Design and Analysis of Bioavailability and Bioequivalence Studies, Second Edition, Revised and Expanded,* Shein-Chung Chow and Jen-pei Liu
4. *Meta-Analysis in Medicine and Health Policy,* Dalene K. Stangl and Donald A. Berry
5. *Generalized Linear Models: A Bayesian Perspective,* Dipak K. Dey, Sujit K. Ghosh, and Bani K. Mallick
6. *Difference Equations with Public Health Applications,* Lemuel A. Moyé and Asha Seth Kapadia
7. *Medical Biostatistics,* Abhaya Indrayan and Sanjeev B. Sarmukaddam
8. *Statistical Methods for Clinical Trials,* Mark X. Norleans
9. *Causal Analysis in Biomedicine and Epidemiology: Based on Minimal Sufficient Causation,* Mikel Aickin
10. *Statistics in Drug Research: Methodologies and Recent Developments,* Shein-Chung Chow and Jun Shao
11. *Sample Size Calculations in Clinical Research,* Shein-Chung Chow, Jun Shao, and Hansheng Wang
12. *Applied Statistical Design for the Researcher,* Daryl S. Paulson
13. *Advances in Clinical Trial Biostatistics,* Nancy L. Geller
14. *Statistics in the Pharmaceutical Industry, Third Edition,* Ralph Buncher and Jia-Yeong Tsay
15. *DNA Microarrays and Related Genomics Techniques: Design, Analysis, and Interpretation of Experiments,* David B. Allsion, Grier P. Page, T. Mark Beasley, and Jode W. Edwards
16. *Basic Statistics and Pharmaceutical Statistical Applications, Second Edition,* James E. De Muth
17. *Adaptive Design Methods in Clinical Trials,* Shein-Chung Chow and Mark Chang
18. *Handbook of Regression and Modeling: Applications for the Clinical and Pharmaceutical Industries,* Daryl S. Paulson
19. *Statistical Design and Analysis of Stability Studies,* Shein-Chung Chow
20. *Sample Size Calculations in Clinical Research, Second Edition,* Shein-Chung Chow, Jun Shao, and Hansheng Wang
21. *Elementary Bayesian Biostatistics,* Lemuel A. Moyé
22. *Adaptive Design Theory and Implementation Using SAS and R,* Mark Chang
23. *Computational Pharmacokinetics,* Anders Källén

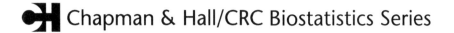
Chapman & Hall/CRC Biostatistics Series

Computational Pharmacokinetics

Anders Källén

AstraZeneca R&D

Lund, Sweden

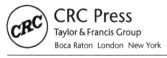

CRC Press

Taylor & Francis Group

Boca Raton London New York

CRC Press is an imprint of the
Taylor & Francis Group, an **informa** business

A CHAPMAN & HALL BOOK

CRC Press
Taylor & Francis Group
6000 Broken Sound Parkway NW, Suite 300
Boca Raton, FL 33487-2742

First issued in paperback 2019

© 2008 by Taylor & Francis Group, LLC
CRC Press is an imprint of Taylor & Francis Group, an Informa business

No claim to original U.S. Government works

ISBN-13: 978-1-4200-6065-2 (hbk)
ISBN-13: 978-0-367-38884-3 (pbk)

Library of Congress Cataloging-in-Publication Data

Källén, Anders.
    Computational pharmacokinetics / Anders Källén.
        p. ; cm. -- (Chapman & Hall/CRC biostatistics series ; 23)
    Includes bibliographical references and index.
    ISBN-13: 978-1-4200-6065-2 (hardcover : alk. paper)
    ISBN-10: 1-4200-6065-1 (hardcover : alk. paper)
    1. Pharmacokinetics--Data processing. I. Title. II. Series.
    [DNLM: 1. Pharmacokinetics--Mathematical models. 2. Empirical Research.
3. Models, Theoretical. QV 38 K137c 2007]

RM301.5.K35 2007
615'.70285--dc22   2007013826

Visit the Taylor & Francis Web site at
http://www.taylorandfrancis.com

and the CRC Press Web site at
http://www.crcpress.com

Anders Källén

Computational
Pharmacokinetics

CRC PRESS
Boca Raton   London   New York   Washington, D.C.

Series Introduction

The primary objectives of the Chapman & Hall/CRC Biostatistics Series are to provide useful reference books for researchers and scientists in academia, industry, and government, and also to offer textbooks for undergraduate and/or graduate courses in the area of biostatistics. This book series will provide comprehensive and unified presentations of statistical designs and analyses of important applications in biostatistics, such as those in biopharmaceuticals. A well-balanced summary will be given of current and recently developed statistical methods and interpretations for both statisticians and researchers/scientists with minimal statistical knowledge, who are engaged in the field of applied biostatistics. The series is committed to providing easy-to-understand, state-of-the-art references and textbooks. In each book, statistical concepts and methodologies will be illustrated through real-world examples.

For a given drug product, it is of interest to study how the drug moves through the body and the processes of movement such as absorption (A), distribution (D), metabolism (M), and excretion (E) after drug administration. The key concept of a pharmacokinetic (PK) study is to study what the body does to the drug (which is usually characterized by ADME of a drug product after administration), while the key concept of a pharmacodynamic (PD) study is to study what the drug does to the body. This leads to the study of PK or population PK. The goal of a PK/PD study is to study the relationship between dose and response, which provides insightful information regarding: (i) how best to choose doses at which to evaluate a drug, (ii) how best to use a drug in a population, and (iii) how best to use a drug to treat individual patients or subpopulations of patients. Unlike most researchers in the area, the author focuses on mathematical models for PK parameters rather than the population PK, which is the application of nonlinear mixed effects modelling to PK models.

This book in the series, *Computational Pharmacokinetics*, provides useful (mathematical model) approaches for PK studies in pharmaceutical research and development. It covers empirical PK, numerical methods for PK parameter estimation, physiological aspects of PK, modelling the distribution process, and PK/PD modelling. It would be beneficial to pharmaceutical scientists/researchers and biostatisticians who are engaged in the areas of pharmaceutical research and development.

Shein-Chung Chow
Editor-in-Chief
Chapman & Hall/CRC Biostatistics Series

Preface

The study of how the body handles various substances, in particular drugs we take, is called pharmacokinetics and started out as an application of linear differential equations. However, as the subject grew in clinical importance, this proved a barrier to learning it and the subject was therefore reformulated in more physiological terms, with the little mathematics that remained considered a nuisance. Today pharmacokinetics plays an important role in the early development of new drugs.

This author started out studying mathematics and encountered pharmacokinetics when joining the pharmaceutical industry. Since then he has nurtured a dream to get the opportunity to show, in particular to statisticians, with a mathematical background, what the subject is about – mathematical modelling. In the summer of 2006 there was an opening, and this book is the result.

It is important to note that this is a book about pharmacokinetics for statisticians, not a book about statistical aspects of pharmacokinetics. It is not a book about methods for model fitting, nonlinear regression or mixed effects models, neither is it a book about statistical models for pharmacokinetic parameters. In particular, there is almost no discussion on the subject of population kinetics, since this is the application of nonlinear mixed effects modelling to pharmacokinetic models.

There are a number of apologies that seems appropriate to do at this stage:

1. There is a very short reference list to this book. I spend far too little time reading scientific articles, and (therefore?) find it better to omit giving credit to people than to give credit to the wrong people. With this approach there is also no risk of claiming originality of any part of the present work by mistake, since none is claimed.

2. This book has been written from the perspective of pharmacokinetics as an area in applied mathematics. This viewpoint may not go down well with many contemporary workers in the field. I hope, however, that the way it has been developed, building on the accepted concepts of the pharmacokinetics of today, can lead to forgiveness at least by some.

Given these apologies, a few words on what has inspired this book might not be amiss. The first inspiration is a delightful book by D.S. Riggs [5] on the mathematical treatise of physiological phenomena. My first non-trivial contact with real-life pharmacokinetics was in a course given by Apotekarsocieten in Sweden in 1988. Among other things, that course directed me to what may be the standard treatise of clinical pharmacokinetics [6], a book deliberately written using very little mathematics. This, of course, is the reason for the success it has had. The final piece of inspiration for me was the one-week workshop which professors Malcolm Rowland and Lewis Sheiner with co-workers have had for many years in *Advanced Methods in Pharmacokinetics and Pharmacodynamics*, and which I attended in 1993. Any overlap between the content of that workshop and the content of this book is definitely not a coincidence.

There is only one real-life example in this book. It is however used extensively and the author wants to thank his employer, AstraZeneca, for allowing the usage of these data without any constraints.

I want to thank a few people for helping me by reviewing and making comments at different stages of the development of this book. Thanks are due to Tore Persson and Eva Bredberg, colleagues at AstraZeneca, to Professor Michael C. Makoid and to my father, Professor Bengt Källén.

Finally, this book was written in LaTeX, and the software used for computations and graphics was the high level matrix programming language GAUSS, distributed by Aptech Systems of Maple Valley, Washington. Most of the code is part of a bigger library of statistical and other GAUSS procedures.

Anders Källén
Lund, March 2007

Contents

Chapter 1

Introduction

1.1 Goal with this book

When you take a drug, you do that because you want an effect – reduced headache, relief from an asthma attack, lower blood pressure, or something else. When you swallow a tablet, the substance in it is absorbed and distributed in the body, before being metabolized and/or eliminated. The science that deals with this is pharmacokinetics, abbreviated PK. It involves a modelling part in which data obtained from clinical studies are used to describe how the drug is handled by and distributed in the body. Clinical pharmacokinetics is the bedside application of this information, assuring that the drug is appropriately used in the treatment of a medical condition.

The subject of pharmacokinetics was born in 1937 when T. Teorell published a two-part paper titled *Kinetics of distribution of substances administered to the body*. In this and subsequent works of others, pharmacokinetics was a description based on compartmental models, which essentially made it into a simple application of the theory of linear differential equations in mathematics. During the 1970's, spearheaded by professor Malcolm Rowland of Manchester University and others, the focus was shifted to more physiological concepts, primarily clearance and volume, which made the information more directly useful to clinicians. With this, the presentation of the subject shifted from a mathematical modelling perspective, which represented a barrier to understanding for many students of the field, towards a concept based largely on a non-mathematical description.

This book is not about the clinical application of pharmacokinetics. It is about the basic concepts and models of pharmacokinetics from a mathematical perspective. It is about the mathematical foundations of the basic pharmacokinetic concepts and the computational aspects around them. It is widely believed that mathematics in some way blurs the true meaning of the basic concepts in pharmacokinetics. This book tries to demonstrate that the opposite is true. It tries to outline pharmacokinetics from the mathematical modelling viewpoint based on clinically relevant PK parameters. There is more to pharmacokinetics than this book addresses. For example, knowledge of the physio-chemical properties of a drug is useful for understanding the basic processes involved: absorption, distribution, metabolism, and elimination (abbreviated ADME). However, chemistry is hardly touched upon in this book. There is no discussion about polarity of molecules or CYP enzymes in the liver and how such information is used.

The primary audience for this book is mathematicians and statisticians who need to analyze this kind of data. Most of the everyday mathematical modelling in pharmacokinetics is made without deep knowledge of the structural properties of substances or human physiology, and this book is about such mathematical modelling. A mathematician/statistician who wants to learn about the more clinical aspects of pharmacokinetics is referred to other literature. On the other hand, this book may also be useful to people with another background, such as experienced pharmacokineticists or even some clinical pharmacologists.

1.2   A short course in pharmacokinetics

In this section we will give an ultra-short overview of pharmacokinetics. The material covered here is expanded on in the rest of this book.

In pharmacokinetics we measure a drug concentration $C(t)$ in some blood compartment. The amount of drug in the body is governed by the equation

$$M'(t) = a(t) - CL(t)C(t), \quad M(0) = 0,$$

where $a(t)$ is the uptake rate and $CL(t)$ is called the clearance. From this an average clearance is obtained:

$$CL_{av} = \frac{\int_0^\infty a(t)\, dt}{\int_0^\infty C(t)\, dt},$$

where the numerator is the total amount of drug absorbed.

When we want to study how a particular drug is distributed within, and eliminated from, the body, it is convenient to get rid of all absorption issues by giving a bolus dose. Giving a bolus dose is equivalent to taking $a(t) = 0$ and $M(0)$ equal to the dose D given. If all drug is eventually eliminated, after a bolus dose, it follows that

$$M(t) = \int_t^\infty CL(s)C(s)\, ds.$$

The fraction $M(t)/D$ can be interpreted as the survival distribution function of a stochastic variable, the time a drug molecule spends in the body. The mean value of this distribution is called the mean residence time of the drug, and is abbreviated MRT.

In the classical non-compartmental description of how the drug is distributed in the body we use the volume $V(t)$ defined by $M(t) = V(t)C(t)$. This is the volume the drug would be distributed in, provided it was well mixed with the same concentration everywhere. In general $V(t)$ is an increasing function, starting from a value V_c which measures the volume of the space we sample from (called the central compartment), and which asymptotically approaches a value V_d, the volume of distribution, as t approaches infinity. $V(t)$ describes the relative distribution of drug between the central space and the rest of the body at time t. Another volume parameter of particular interest is the volume in steady state, defined by $V_{ss} = \mathrm{MRT} \cdot CL_{av}$, which measures the volume when we balance elimination exactly by adding new drug to the system.

Most drugs are not well mixed in the body. There are various physiological processes which affect drug molecules: these are transported around the body in the blood, often bound to special proteins, and free drug escapes into different tissues with different physiological characteristics and gets bound to proteins there. What happens to the drug in the body can be visualized by considering the body as being made up of a (very) large number of compartments, each of which has a well-defined volume in which the drug is well mixed. Drug is then transferred between these compartments, either transported by the blood from one to another, or by passing an interior membrane in some body organ. A compartment can also be a biochemical transformation of the drug in some space. The drug is eliminated from some compartments, the most important examples being (irreversible) metabolic conversion in liver cells and excretion in the kidneys. In all we can visualize this whole process as a dynamic system described by a system of ordinary differential equations of the form

$$C'(t) = AC(t)$$

where $C(t)$ is a vector of concentrations in the different compartments. The coefficient matrix A describes how different compartments are connected. These coefficients need not be constants. If one or more of them are functions of compartment concentrations we have a non-linear PK system. If they are independent of concentrations but still time-dependent, we have a time-dependent PK system (also called *chrono-pharmacokinetics*). When all coefficients in A are constants we have a linear PK system. Intuitively this is equivalent to an assumption that the histories of different drug molecules in the body are independent of each other, so that there is no competition for some enzyme or transport process.

It is out of the question to describe in detail what the PK system for a particular drug looks like, based on only the observed concentrations $C(t)$ in the central compartment. However, one can try to build models that capture the essentials by lumping together similar physiological spaces (in a wide sense) and thereby reducing the number of compartments. The crudest such division is to divide the body into two spaces, the central from which we sample, and a peripheral space, about which we get no first-hand information. Then we can make more or less complicated assumptions about the peripheral space, leading up to so-called compartmental models which are systems of ordinary differential equations with constant coefficients. In doing that, however, there are identification problems and one typically needs to make non-verifiable assumptions in order to be able to identify and characterize the unknowns of such a model.

An alternative to build compartmental models is to approach the problem of describing the distribution from the perspective of what we see in the central compartment. Let us assume that the flow from the central space to the peripheral space is proportional to the concentration in the central space, whereas the return flow depends on the history of $C(t)$ (because the time drug molecules spend in the peripheral space before returning differ). This can be expressed as

$$V_c C'(t) = (h * C)(t) - CL_d C(t) - CL_c(t)C(t),$$

where CL_d is called the distributional clearance and $CL_c(t)$ is a clearance function for elimination from the central space. By determining the function $h(t)$ we get a description of how drug passes through the peripheral space. From it we can define, for instance, a parameter describing the mean transit time of the peripheral space for a drug molecule as

$$\text{MTT}_p = \frac{\int_0^\infty th(t)\,dt}{\int_0^\infty h(t)\,dt}.$$

Compartmental models correspond to $h(t)$ being sums of exponential functions.

In order to study the input function $a(t)$ we study PK systems that are linear. Then there is a basic relationship between $C(t)$ and the concentration $G(t)$ after a unit bolus dose, namely

$$C(t) = \int_0^t G(t-s)a(s)\,ds.$$

This equation describes the concentration as the result of the process of absorption followed by the process of distribution and elimination. By appropriately designed experiments, this allows us to reconstruct the drug uptake function $a(t)$ for a swallowed tablet.

When multiple doses are given at fixed time intervals of length τ, one eventually arrives a τ-periodic steady state concentration $C_{ss}(t)$ over a dosing interval, the interval between two consecutive doses. Steady state here refers to the fact that consecutive doses produce identical concentration profiles. For $C_{ss}(t)$, where t is the time since last dose, we have the simple relation

$$C_{ss}(t) = C(t) + C_{ss}(t+\tau),$$

where τ is the time between two consecutive doses. The second term on the right is the residual concentration of all but the last dose. From this simple relation we can derive various relations between the single-dose concentration $C(t)$ and the steady state concentration $C_{ss}(t)$, relations which are useful when we want to predict from a single dose administration what happens after multiple doses.

The science in which we measure the drug's effect $E(t)$ over time, instead of blood concentrations, is called pharmacodynamics, abbreviated PD. Models that attempt to predict $E(t)$ from blood concentrations $C(t)$ are called PK/PD models. If we hold the concentration fixed and measure the effect in equilibrium we get a relation $E = \Phi(C)$, for what is typically an increasing function of sigmoidal shape. However, if we are not studying the system in equilibrium, there is typically a delay between changes in $C(t)$ and changes in $E(t)$. One way to reduce it to the functional relation given by Φ is to assume that the effect is not a direct function of concentration, but of its history up to that time. This means that we assume $E = \Phi(H * C)$ for some function $H(t)$, a modelling approach that is called the biophase method. Alternatively we can model the delay between concentration and effect by making some assumptions on the dynamics of $E(t)$. The latter approach may be relevant when the effect we measure is the concentration of some substance which occurs naturally in the body. Such substances may be modelled by a turn-over model in which

$$E'(t) = k_{in}(t) - k_{out}E(t),$$

where the drug under investigation could affect either of the production rate $k_{in}(t)$ or the degradation rate constant k_{out}.

This was an ultra-short description of some key areas we are going to describe in more detail in the rest of the book. The next section describes how the book is organized.

1.3 Overview of book disposition

Here is a short summary of the book. We start with a focus on the basic empirical pharmacokinetics, including fundamental concepts like clearance and volume. These concepts are derived from simple mass-balance considerations, expressed as mathematical equations. Most of the chapter focusses on what is called the non-compartmental approach to pharmacokinetics. First we discuss distribution and elimination as events after a bolus dose, after which we incorporate an absorption process to discuss both single and multiple dosing of formulations of the drug. Most of the discussion is around linear PK systems, but we also discuss a simple pharmacokinetics system with a capacity limited elimination process. In such a system the basic PK parameters behave differently at an increase of the dose given as compared to the simple behavior for the linear systems, discussed in the non-compartmental approach. We end that chapter by considering an alternative modelling approach, focussed on the fact that the drug is transported around in the body by the blood, instead of using volumes as the basic concepts.

Chapter 3 is about number crunching, i.e., analysis of PK data. First we look at how integrals are estimated from the type of data obtained in pharmacokinetics, as well as the determination of the terminal elimination rate and how to derive a description of an absorption process through numerical deconvolution. Thereafter we work our way through a set of real-life data, in which two inhaled steroids are compared from a pharmacokinetics point of view. This is an elaborate example of most aspects of what has been discussed up to that point. The chapter ends with a very short discussion on how pharmacokinetics typically is studied in a drug development project.

In Chapter 4 we take a rather short tour through some physiological aspects of pharmacokinetics, mainly because it helps us to understand some of the concepts that were defined and analyzed up to that point. In this chapter, we will get a better understanding of PK volumes and we will build a simple physiological model for an imagined drug. We will also analyze this physiological model with the methods discussed in the previous two chapters in order to see how their outcomes compare to the actual model. We also discuss some aspects of the processes involved when a tablet is dissolved in the intestines in order to be absorbed.

In Chapter 5 we take a deeper look into how to describe the distribution aspect of pharmacokinetics. We introduce compartmental models, show their limitations and finally build a general-purpose type of model which is fitted to the amount of information we actually have from plasma. This is essentially an extension of the non-compartmental modelling approach that is discussed in Chapter 2. Both the model per se and how to analyze it numerically is discussed, and we apply the methods to the steroid data discussed in Chapter 3.

In the last chapter, we make a few comments about the relationship between drug concentration and effect, so-called PK/PD modelling. So much is known about the biology of parts of this, that it is important to point out that the approach we take is one of generality. We only describe dynamic principles from a mathematical perspective.

Even though the primary audience of this book is people with a basic mathematical background, attempts have been made to describe most of the formulas in words; most mathematical derivations that are more than a few lines have been put in special boxes, in order not disrupt the general flow of the discussion. That is not to say that the discussion in any way is easy to follow without basic mathematical training.

For the remainder of this introductory chapter we will briefly discuss a few preparatory items that will be useful in later chapters. You may skip these sections, or only read them superficially, and then return to them if necessary when reading later chapters. If you are a pharmacokineticist by training, you should however read at least the first few paragraphs in the next section, where some notation is discussed.

1.4 Integrals and convolution

In this section we introduce some notation that will be used repeatedly in what follows.

First and foremost we will use the two operators

I(.): which is simply the integral

$$I(f) = \int_0^\infty f(t)\, dt.$$

E(.):

$$E(f) = \int_0^\infty t f(t)\, dt,$$

which is often called the first moment.

This notation will be used interchanged with explicitly writing out the integrals in question. All integrals are assumed to converge. If $f(t)$ is a probability density function, then $E(f)$ is its expected value, but we use the notation more in a more general way. However it will be a common feature that we, for non-negative functions $f(t)$ defined for $t \geq 0$, will interpret the ratio $E(f)/I(f)$ as the mean value of some stochastic time variable.

Geometrically $I(f)$ is the area between the t-axis and the curve defined by the function $f(t)$, and in pharmacokinetics such integrals are therefore called the *Area Under the Curve* and denoted AUC. Also, in pharmacokinetics, $E(f)$ is usually called the *Area Under the Moment Curve* and denoted AUMC. We will not use this notation because we need to be able to specify in the notation which function we integrate.

Simple but useful properties of the integral and the first moment are

$$I(f') = -f(0), \quad E(f') = -I(f). \tag{1.1}$$

For two functions $f(t), g(t)$, both defined for $t \geq 0$, we define their *convolution* by

$$(f * g)(t) = \int_0^t f(t - s) g(s) ds. \tag{1.2}$$

It is a commutative operation, in that $(f * g)(t) = (g * f)(t)$. It is also associative:

$$((f * g) * h)(t) = (f * (g * h))(t).$$

To facilitate future discussions, we will collect some properties of the convolution operator here.

First we note that the convolution of two exponential functions $f(t) = e^{-at}$ and $g(t) = e^{-bt}$ is given by, if $a \neq b$,

$$e^{-at} * e^{-bt} = e^{-at} \int_0^t e^{(a-b)s} ds = \frac{1}{a-b}(e^{-bt} - e^{-at}). \qquad (1.3)$$

If $a = b$ the convolution is te^{-at}.

In general, we have for integration that

$$I(f * g) = I(f)I(g), \qquad (1.4)$$

because

$$\int_0^\infty \int_0^t f(t-s)g(s)dsdt = \int_0^\infty \left(\int_s^\infty f(t-s)dt\right)g(s)ds =$$

$$\left(\int_0^\infty f(t)dt\right)\left(\int_0^\infty g(s)ds\right),$$

and for the expected value we have that

$$E(f * g) = I(f)E(g) + E(f)I(g), \qquad (1.5)$$

which is derived in a completely analogous way. Formulae 1.4 and 1.5 will be used repeatedly in what follows. One direct consequence of Equations 1.4 and 1.5 is that

$$\frac{E(f * g)}{I(f * g)} = \frac{E(f)}{I(f)} + \frac{E(g)}{I(g)},$$

a formula that corresponds to the well-known statement in probability theory that the mean of the sum of two stochastic variables is the sum of the means of these.

If we differentiate formula 1.2 with respect to t, we get

$$(f * g)'(t) = f(0)g(t) + (f' * g)(t). \qquad (1.6)$$

Applying this to the function

$$F(t) = \int_t^\infty f(s)ds$$

instead of $f(t)$, we find that $(F * g)'(t) = I(f)g(t) - (f * g)(t)$, since $F'(t) = -f(t)$ and $F(0) = I(f)$. It follows that

$$\int_t^\infty (f * g)(s)ds = (F * g)(t) + I(f) \int_t^\infty g(s)ds. \qquad (1.7)$$

Solving the convolution equation $h = f * g$ for $f(t)$, when $h(t)$ and $g(t)$ are known, is called *deconvolution*.

1.5 Linear kinetics and compartments

There are two concepts that will be used extensively in the coming chapters, but are not well defined there. These concepts are a *linear PK system* and *compartment*. In this section we will give a preliminary discussion on the meaning of these concepts, which the reader can skip on first reading.

By a *system* we mean a map that takes an input function $f(t)$ to an output function $h(t)$. Denote such a map $h = T(f)$. It is linear if the condition $T(af_1 + bf_2) = aT(f_1) + bT(f_2)$ holds (all continuity conditions are taken for granted) and can be written in the form

$$T(f)(t) = \int_{-\infty}^{\infty} K(t,s)f(s)\,ds.$$

In a PK system, t is a time variable starting at $t = 0$, and there is a time causality which assumes that values $f(s)$ for $s > t$ cannot influence the value of $T(f)(t)$. Thus the function $K(t,s)$ is assumed to fulfill $K(t,s) = 0$ when $s > t$. So, for a PK system the output function $h(t)$ and the input function $f(t)$ are related through

$$h(t) = \int_0^t K(t,s)f(s)\,ds$$

for a kernel function $K(t,s)$. When a PK system is described in this way, it is a time-dependent PK system. To be a linear PK system, it also needs to be time homogeneous so that the function $K(t,s)$ takes the form $K(t-s)$. This means that $h = K * f$.

The equation

$$h(t) = \int_0^t K(t-s)f(s)\,ds$$

is often called a *transport equation* and appears repeatedly in pharmacokinetics. Note that if $f(t) = \delta_0$ is the unit impulse at time 0 (the Dirac measure) the output function $h(t)$ of the system is the kernel function $K(t)$.

The word compartment as used in this book refers in general to a fluid space with a hypothetical volume within which we can assume the drug we study to be well mixed so that it gets a well-defined concentration. It also includes the possibility of a bio-transformed version of the drug.

In Chapter 5 we discuss compartmental *models*. What is generally called compartmental models in pharmacokinetics should probably better be called linear state models: the drug under investigation enters and exits different states, which may be physical spaces or biochemical transformations of the drug. In these models, a key feature is that the exit rate from the state is proportional to the amount in it. In the body, the driving force for processes in general is local, so that it is not the total amount that determines the rate of a transport, but the local concentration. Mathematically this means that a compartmental model with q compartment is described by a q-(column)vector $M(t) = (M_1(t), \ldots, M_q(t))$, where $M_i(t)$ is the amount of drug in compartment i at time t. Assuming we give a bolus dose $D = (D_1, \ldots, D_q)$, where D_i is the dose given to compartment i, $M(t)$ is governed by a differential equation

$$M'(t) = AM(t), \quad M(0) = D, \tag{1.8}$$

where A is a $q \times q$ matrix with elements $q_{ij} \geq 0, i \neq j$ and $q_{ii} \leq 0$.

However, if we build a model of compartments but assume at least one of the processes that transports the drug between them to be capacity limited, we do not have a compartmental model. This amounts to allowing some coefficients of A to be time dependent, possibly by being a function of components of $M(t)$. In general it is reasonable to assume that the rate out of a particular compartment i depends only on $M_i(t)$, and not the other components. In fact, most biological processes are expected to be local, so they are driven by the local concentration, not the total amount. For that reason we may want to introduce volumes of the compartments, which in turn gives us a concentration $C_i(t)$ in each compartment. We can then redefine our coefficient matrix A so that equation 1.8 is valid for concentrations instead.

When A is a matrix of constants, the solution to equation 1.8 can be written $M(t) = e^{-At}D$. If we replace the bolus dose with a vector function $a(t)$ whose component $a_i(t)$ describes the rate of external drug input to compartment i, we instead get the equation

$$M'(t) = a(t) + AM(t), \quad M(0) = 0,$$

for which the solution can be written

$$M(t) = \int_0^t e^{-A(t-s)} a(s) \, ds.$$

The concept of a linear PK system is very much related to a drug kinetics described by time-independent rate constants.

1.6   Markov processes and compartmental models

If we add one compartment to our compartmental model, containing the cumulative amount of drug $M_{q+1}(t)$ which has been eliminated at time t, and redefine equation 1.8 (adding M_{q+1} to the vector M, the appropriate row to A and a last component 0 to D), we get a version of equation 1.8 which (essentially) describes a time-continuous Markov process with an absorbing state (the last one). In fact, divide $M(t)$ with $\sum_i D_i$, and equation 1.8 becomes Kolmogorov's forward equation for such a system.

It is natural that we should be able to interpret a compartmental model as a stochastic process. A bolus dose consists of a very large number of molecules, and these will transit the different compartments in different ways. If we focus on an individual drug molecule, all we can make claims about is the probability that it goes here or there. In fact, what the interpretation of equation 1.8 as a Markov process says, is that a drug molecule in state i at time t will have, in a very short time interval h, a probability of $q_{ij}h$ of going to state $j \neq i$. It also means that the time a particular drug molecule spends in compartment i is exponentially distributed with mean $-1/q_{ii}$.

Much of this remains true if we allow the rate constants to depend on the concentration in the compartment. We can define a Markov process with density dependent rate constants similar to as we did above. Now the waiting time need not be exponential, but equation 1.8 will be a valid description of the amount of drug in the different compartments, interpreted as an expected value.

In the coming discussion on pharmacokinetics, there is always an underlying probability model which can be assumed to be a Markov process. We will not state it explicitly anywhere, but will use the concept of mean transit times and mean residence times in different spaces. These are expected values of some distributions that describe the transit time and residence time of a drug molecule in the space in question. Hopefully the mixture between the mainly deterministic approach and the particular probabilistic interpretation will not present a problem.

Chapter 2

Empirical pharmacokinetics

2.1 Problem specification and some notations

In this chapter, we are going to discuss the standard model (or description) of pharmacokinetics. It is a description where elimination is expressed in terms of clearance (the volume cleared of drug per time unit) and in which distribution is expressed in terms of volumes. The basis of this description is a simple mass-balance equation. Before we can write it down, however, we need some notation:

$M(t)$: The amount of drug in the body at time t. It is generally expressed as number of molecules (moles) or mass (weight).

$a(t)$: The rate at which the drug enters the body at time t. It is generally expressed as moles/time unit or mass/time unit.

$e(t)$: The rate at which the drug disappears from the body at time t. It has the same unit as $a(t)$.

With this notation we have a basic mass balance equation

$$M'(t) = a(t) - e(t), \tag{2.1}$$

i.e., the rate of change of mass equals the rate in minus the rate out.

One consequence of this is that

$$\int_0^\infty e(t)dt = M(0) + \int_0^\infty a(t)dt - M(\infty),$$

where we interpret the right-hand-side as the amount of drug, D, that ever is seen in blood minus what is never eliminated.

As such this equation is not very useful; none of its components are directly measurable. In fact, what we can measure is typically only

$C(t)$ the concentration of drug in some blood compartment, like whole blood, serum or plasma. If not otherwise stated, we will assume that our drug concentrations are measured in plasma.

Sometimes we may supplement this measurement with measurements in urine. In such a case we collect urine over a certain period $[t_1, t_2]$ and measure drug concentration in that sample. Since we know the volume of the sample we can calculate the amount of drug in the portion, i.e., the amount excreted through the kidneys in the time interval $[t_1, t_2]$ (though there is usually a small amount left in the bladder when urination is completed). For special drugs there are also other compartments where we can measure, like the cerebrospinal liquor.

Typically, therefore, our problem is to derive as much information as possible about how the molecules are handled by the body from only plasma concentrations.

Note that the body is not a container in which the drug is homogeneously mixed. The drug is transported around the body by the blood, from which it leaves and enters various tissues, from which it is eliminated or later returned to the blood. Within the plasma we may assume that the drug is well mixed, so that there is a meaningful concentration $C(t)$ in that at time t. But there may be a considerable amount of drug elsewhere in the body, drug we cannot measure directly.

2.2   Distribution and elimination

2.2.1   Linear kinetics and bolus dose

Distribution and elimination are processes that can be intricate and involve capacity limited processes. If that is the case, the fate of a particular drug molecule depends on the presence or absence of other molecules (these may, for instance, block a saturable pathway) and its behavior may therefore be different than to what it would have been, had it been on its own. Systems for which this does not happen are called *linear PK systems* if they also are time homogeneous. For such systems we have that if we give a unit dose and get plasma concentration $C(t)$, giving a dose D in the same way at time s would give us the plasma concentration $DC(t - s)$ at time t.

For linear PK systems a number of general statements can be made which justifies what is called the Non-Compartmental Approach (NCA) to data analysis, which is the focus of this chapter. This approach to PK analysis is independent on any assumptions on compartment models, as introduced in Section 1.5 and more fully discussed in Chapter 5, and therefore often considered model free. But it hinges on the assumption of a linear PK system. If we have a non-linear system, like one in which the elimination process is capacity limited, we may have to go back to the original mass-balance equations in order to obtain useful information. For some further discussion on this see, see Section 2.5.

When studying distribution and elimination, this is best done by studying plasma concentrations obtained after what is called a bolus dose. This means that, when we start our clock, the dose we give, D, is mixed in a space containing plasma, providing us with a start concentration. This is an ideal state, corresponding to the use of the Dirac measure in other applications of mathematics. Most of the discussion on distribution and elimination which follows assumes that we have given a bolus dose.

In real life the closest we can get to a bolus dose is to give an intravenous shot of the drug. In reality that means that we have at time zero a localized amount of drug which is transported through the blood vessels. It soon gets mixed in plasma, but it takes a few circulations through the blood vessel system before it can actually be considered evenly mixed and provides a well defined plasma concentration. And in the meantime some of it may have left the blood vessels for other parts of the body. So the start concentration $C(0)$ we discuss above is not a real concentration; it is a mathematical abstraction which will be determined by backward extrapolation from later observations.

When a bolus dose is given, the volume the drug is distributed in includes plasma but is often larger. This defines a (theoretical) volume of the body in which the drug has the same concentration as in the plasma. We call that part of the body the *central compartment* and denote its volume V_c. In particular it means that (with a bolus dose)

$$D = C(0)V_c.$$

2.2.2 Clearance

The plasma clearance function $CL(t)$ is defined as the proportionality factor

$$e(t) = CL(t)C(t).$$

Thus $CL(t)$ is the rate at which plasma is cleared of drug and has the unit volume per time unit – like a flow. We will always assume that this function has a limit, $CL(\infty)$, which it rapidly approaches as $t \to \infty$. The fundamental equation 2.1 is now rewritten as

$$M'(t) = a(t) - CL(t)C(t). \tag{2.2}$$

An immediate consequence of this is the fundamental relation between the dose D that enters the body and the plasma clearance:

$$D = \int_0^\infty CL(t)C(t)\,dt. \tag{2.3}$$

We have here made the assumption that all drug is eventually eliminated. Note that this relation is independent of how the drug was given, as long as it is eventually eliminated and D represents the amount of drug that is ever observed in the blood stream. If we control the dose that appears at the site of measurement, we can compute an average plasma clearance

$$CL_{av} = \frac{D}{\int_0^\infty C(t)\,dt}. \tag{2.4}$$

In many situations a reasonable assumption to make is that plasma clearance is time-independent, and $CL(t)$ therefore a constant. If clearance is constant, formula 2.4 tells us how to compute it from the plasma concentrations. In Chapter 5 we will see that this assumption means that elimination of drug is from the central compartment, which for most linear PK system is a reasonable approximation. A situation where clearance is time-dependent is when it is a function of the drug concentration. As an example, a capacity limited elimination process can often be modelled by

$$CL(t) = \frac{A}{B + C(t)}$$

for some constants A and B. For practical purposes such a clearance is constant if $C(t) << B$, and constant clearance is a desirable property. The most important example of non-linearity is when the elimination is through metabolic conversion in the liver by enzymes that are not very abundant. Some aspects of this case will be discussed further in Section 2.5. We refer to the part of clearance that is due to metabolic conversion as the metabolic clearance of the drug, and denote it CL_M.

Another route of elimination is excretion with the urine. If $U(t)$ denotes the amount of drug excreted into the urine in the interval $[0, t]$, we define the renal clearance as the proportionality constant $CL_R(t)$ in

$$U'(t) = CL_R(t)C(t), \tag{2.5}$$

where $U'(t)$ is the rate of elimination through the kidneys. If we collect urine over the interval $[t_1, t_2]$ we get an average renal clearance over that interval by integrating equation 2.5:

$$CL_R = \frac{U(t_2) - U(t_1)}{\int_{t_1}^{t_2} C(t)\,dt}.$$

If we make the urine sampling long enough, we can also estimate the total amount of drug excreted, $U(\infty)$, and the fraction excreted

$$f_e = \frac{U(\infty)}{D}.$$

Note that the average renal excretion over the whole interval is

$$CL_R = \frac{U(\infty)}{D} \frac{D}{\int_0^\infty C(t)\,dt} = f_e CL_{av}.$$

Most drugs are eliminated either by enzymatic breakdown in the liver or excretion by the kidneys. If these are the only two elimination pathways, we can write the total clearance as the sum of a metabolic clearance CL_M and a renal clearance CL_R. The reason it is a sum is anatomical and will be discussed in Chapter 4.

We leave this subsection with the bolus equation, on which we will base much of the following discussion:

$$M'(t) = -CL(t)C(t), \quad M(0) = D. \tag{2.6}$$

2.2.3 Mean residence time and half-life

The function $T_{1/2}(t)$ defined by

$$C(t + T_{1/2}(t)) = C(t)/2$$

measures the time it takes to halve the plasma concentration we have at time t. As $t \to \infty$ this often approaches a limit, $T_{1/2}(t) \to t_{1/2}$, a limit $t_{1/2}$ called the *terminal elimination half-life*. Its existence means that, for large t,

$$C(t) \approx C_0 e^{-\lambda_{el}t}, \quad \lambda_{el} = \frac{\ln 2}{t_{1/2}}.$$

If we plot $\ln C(t)$ versus t, this will for large t look approximately like a straight line for which the negative slope equals λ_{el}, *the terminal elimination rate*.

The terminal elimination rate tells us how quickly the last remnants of drug in the body disappear from plasma. It typically tells us nothing about how long it takes from dosing until the drug is eliminated. We can describe that in terms of a stochastic variable T, which is the time it takes for an individual drug molecule to get eliminated. Its distribution function is derived from the observation that

$$P(T > t) = \{\text{fraction of drug remaining at time } t\} = \frac{M(t)}{D}.$$

The expected value of T is called the *Mean Residence Time* and defined by

$$\text{MRT} = D^{-1} \int_0^\infty t\,(-M'(t))\,dt = D^{-1} \int_0^\infty t\,CL(t)C(t)\,dt, \tag{2.7}$$

or, equivalently,

$$\text{MRT} = \frac{\int_0^\infty t\,CL(t)C(t)\,dt}{\int_0^\infty CL(t)C(t)\,dt}.$$

MRT tells us the average time a drug molecule resides in the body until it is eliminated. In the special case when clearance is constant, we can cancel it out from the expression, and then MRT is the same as the apparent MRT defined by

$$\text{MRT}_{app} = \frac{\int_0^\infty t\,C(t)\,dt}{\int_0^\infty C(t)\,dt}, \tag{2.8}$$

which we can compute from the observed plasma concentration curve. In what follows it is important to distinguish between MRT, which is the true mean residence time, and MRT_{app} which is a computable number from plasma concentrations. The latter can also be computed when the administration is not a bolus dose, but it is only when it is a bolus dose that it estimates the true mean residence time. The relationship between MRT and MRT_{app} will be further discussed later in this book.

In the notational jungle around MRT, let us introduce one further notation. We let MRT_{iv} stand for the apparent MRT after a bolus dose. Thus MRT_{iv} is an approximation of the true MRT. The notation MRT_{app} is used for formula 2.8, irrespective of how dosing was done.

We can proceed, and define higher moments of the distribution as well, like the variance and its apparent version

$$\mathrm{VRT}_{app} = \frac{\int_0^\infty (t - \mathrm{MRT}_{app})^2 C(t)\, dt}{\int_0^\infty C(t)\, dt},$$

but that is not much used, and we do not discuss it further.

2.2.4 Volumes of distributions

In the standard model for pharmacokinetics the extent of distribution of the drug is described in terms of volumes. Volume is here defined as a simple proportionality constant between amount in the body and concentration in plasma:

$$M(t) = V(t)C(t),$$

so it is not immediately clear what it physically means. Numerically these volumes can be hundreds of liters, despite the fact that body water is only about 42 liters. So it is not to be interpreted as a true volume. How to interpret it physiologically is one of the key subjects of Chapter 4.

But the definition of $V(t)$ means that it can be computed. In fact, if we integrate equation 2.6 we find that

$$V(t) = \frac{\int_t^\infty CL(s)C(s)ds}{C(t)}. \tag{2.9}$$

Note that

$$V(0) = D/C(0) = V_c$$

is the volume of the central compartment.

For large t we can assume that $C(t) \approx C_0 e^{-\lambda_{el}t}$ and then

$$V(t) \approx \frac{CL(\infty)C_0 e^{-\lambda_{el}t}/\lambda_{el}}{C_0 e^{-\lambda_{el}t}} = \frac{CL(\infty)}{\lambda_{el}}.$$

This motivates the definition of the (terminal) *volume of distribution* by

$$V_d = \frac{CL}{\lambda_{el}} = \frac{CL \cdot t_{1/2}}{\ln 2}.\qquad(2.10)$$

When defining this number, the clearance used is CL_{av}. If clearance is constant we have that

$$V(t) \to V_d \qquad \text{as } t \to \infty.$$

Please note that the basic parameters here are clearance and volume, from which the terminal behavior, in particular the elimination rate constant, is a consequence.

There is another, more popular volume concept, one not related to a bolus dose, but instead to a constant infusion. A constant infusion of rate $a(t) = R$ leads to a constant plasma concentration C_{ss} and since there is no net uptake or elimination of drug, equation 2.2 tells us that

$$R = CL \cdot C_{ss},$$

at least if clearance is constant. Moreover, the amount of drug M_{ss} in the body under these circumstances is given by $M_{ss} = R \cdot \text{MRT}$, so we find that

$$V_{ss} = \frac{M_{ss}}{C_{ss}} = CL \cdot \text{MRT}.\qquad(2.11)$$

This volume is called the *volume in steady state*. Its strict definition is

$$V_{ss} = CL_{av} \cdot \text{MRT},$$

where MRT is the true, not apparent, mean residence time.

2.2.5 Illustration of non-compartmental PK analysis

Table 2.1 summarizes the basic PK parameters describing distribution and elimination in the NCA approach to data. It assumes that we have given a bolus dose of size D and that we have estimated the terminal elimination rate λ_{el}. Note that in the non-compartmental approach to analysis, the real MRT is taken to be the apparent MRT_{app} and clearance is taken to be the average clearance CL_{av}.

Many plasma concentration curves after a bolus dose can be well approximated with polyexponential functions

$$C(t) = \sum_{k=1}^{c} A_k e^{-\lambda_k t}.$$

The reason for this will be apparent in Chapter 5, but they highlight one feature of distribution and elimination of a typical drug: there are different

Table 2.1: Notation and formulas for the basic pharmacokinetics parameters in non-compartmental analysis

Parameter	Notation	Formula
Terminal half-life:	$t_{1/2}$	$\ln(2)/\lambda_{el}$
Clearance:	CL	$D/\int_0^\infty C(t)dt$
Mean Residence Time:	MRT	$\int_0^\infty t\,C(t)\,dt/\int_0^\infty C(t)\,dt$
Distribution volume:	V_d	CL/λ_{el}
Volume in steady state:	V_{ss}	$CL{\cdot}\text{MRT}$

phases in it. Each such phase is described by a term of the form $Ae^{-\lambda t}$, and different drugs have different number of phases, depending on how complicated their distribution process is. Note that λ_{el} is the smallest of the exponentials λ_k.

One convenient aspect of polyexponentials is that their integrals are easy to compute:

$$\int_0^\infty C(t)dt = \sum_{k=1}^c \frac{A_k}{\lambda_k}, \qquad \int_0^\infty tC(t)dt = \sum_{k=1}^c \frac{A_k}{\lambda_k^2}$$

Here is an illustration of what we have discussed so far.

Example 2.1
A bolus dose of $D = 10$ mg was given of a certain drug, resulting in a plasma concentration profile (unit mg/L) which was well described by the function (time is measured in hours)

$$C(t) = 0.38e^{-1.65t} + 0.18e^{-0.182t}.$$

We will compute the basic PK parameters from this.

The first thing to note is that $C(0) = 0.38 + 0.18 = 0.56$ and since this is equal to D/V_c we see that $V_c = D/C(0) = 17.9$ liters. Also, the terminal half-life is $\ln(2)/0.182 = 3.8$ hours. Using the formulas above we find that

$$\int_0^\infty C(t)dt = 1.22, \qquad \int_0^\infty tC(t)dt = 5.57,$$

from which we deduce that the clearance is $CL = 10/1.22 = 8.20$ L/h and that the (apparent) mean residence time is MRT= $5.57/1.22 = 4.57$ hours. Furthermore, the volume in steady state is estimated to $V_{ss} = 8.20{\cdot}4.57 = 37.5$ liters and the distributional volume to $V_d = 8.20/0.182 = 45.1$ liters.

Figure 2.1 shows in the left subplot the plasma concentration curve on log-scale (solid curve). It illustrates that the later part (after approximately 3

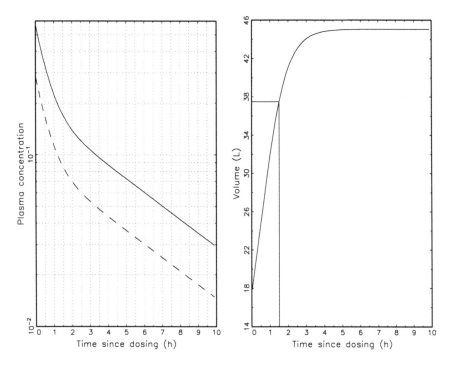

FIGURE 2.1: Plasma concentrations $C(t)$ and volume curve of example. To the left, plasma concentration on log-scale, to the right, volume as a function of time. V_{ss} is marked with lines. For more details, see the text.

hours) is more or less a straight line. The slope of this line gives the terminal elimination rate λ_{el} (in this case 0.182). The dashed curve shows $C(t)/2$, on log-scale, and the horizontal distance between these curves as a function of the left endpoint represents the instantaneous half-life $T_{1/2}(t)$ described above. We see that, e.g., $T_{1/2}(0.5)$ is short, about one hour, whereas as time progresses, the curves become parallel with a distance of 3.8 hours. This is the terminal elimination half-life.

To the right in Figure 2.1, $V(t)$ is plotted using formula 2.9 and the observation that

$$\int_t^\infty Ae^{-\lambda t}\,dt = \frac{A}{\lambda}e^{-\lambda t}.$$

We see that $V(t)$ starts at $V_c = 17.9$ liters and increases asymptotically to $V_d = 45.1$ liters. On the curve $V_{ss} = 37.5$ is marked, a volume obtained after about 1.5 hours.

This example will be further elaborated in Example 5.1, where it will be expressed as a two-compartment model. There we will also learn what V_{ss} means "physiologically" in this case. ⬚

2.3   Absorption

2.3.1   A convolution equation and its consequences

To go beyond the mathematical concept of a bolus dose and study more realistic ways of getting a drug into the body, we go back to the fundamental equation 2.2, which contains the absorption rate $a(t)$ into the central space. Even though we need to return to basics, i.e., equation 2.2, when we study non-linear kinetics, assuming a linear PK system will open up a different angle of approach within the NCA constraints.

So, unless otherwise stated, we assume that the PK is linear. Under that assumption, if the uptake rate of the drug is given by $a(t)$, then the plasma concentration is obtained from the convolution equation

$$C(t) = \int_0^t G(t-s)a(s)\,ds = (G*a)(t), \qquad (2.12)$$

where $G(t)$ is the plasma concentrations obtained after a unit bolus dose. An independent derivation of equation 2.12 is shown in Box 2.1. This fundamental equation tells us all we need to know about absorption, provided we can measure $G(t)$ directly or indirectly. Here is a short summary of key consequences of equation 2.12.

First we apply $I(.)$ (i.e., integrate) to equation 2.12 to get

$$I(C) = I(G)I(a) \iff D = \frac{\int_0^\infty C(t)\,dt}{\int_0^\infty G(t)\,dt}$$

which gives us a formula for how to compute the dose D actually absorbed (as opposed to given). Divided by the dose given, we obtain a fraction F, called the *absolute bioavailability*. If all drug given is absorbed we have $F = 1$, but for various reasons this may not be the case, as discussed later.

Next we apply $E(.)$ to equation 2.12 to get

$$E(C) = I(G)E(a) + E(G)I(a) \iff \frac{E(C)}{I(C)} = \frac{E(G)}{I(G)} + \frac{E(a)}{I(a)}.$$

The entity $E(C)/I(C)$ on the left is the MRT$_{app}$ in the whole body (including the site of administration of the drug, like the gut if we swallow a tablet); the first term on the right hand side is the apparent mean residence time, MRT$_{iv}$, of a bolus dose of the drug, whereas the second term is called the Mean Absorption Time (MAT):

$$\mathrm{MAT} = \frac{\int_0^\infty t\,a(t)\,dt}{\int_0^\infty a(t)\,dt}.$$

Box 2.1 Direct derivation of the convolution equation

We will here do a derivation of equation 2.12 from first principles, in order to highlight the underlying assumptions. Concentrations are assumed to be given in mg/L.

Assume that we give a unit bolus dose at time s, the plasma concentration at time $t > s$ is given by $G(t, s)$. The mathematical linearity of the system then implies that if the dose instead is D mg, the plasma concentration at time t is $DG(t, s)$. Consider a small interval $(s, s + \Delta s)$, during which there is approximately $a(s)\Delta s$ mg of drug absorbed. Its contribution to $C(t)$ is then given by $G(t, s)a(s)\Delta s$, and the assumption of linearity means that in order to obtain the full $C(t)$ we sum such contributions. If we let $\Delta s \to 0$, we get the equation

$$C(t) = \int_0^t G(t, s)a(s)\,ds$$

in the limit. To obtain equation 2.12 we add the other assumption on a linear PK system – that it is homogeneous in time. This means that in order to obtain the contribution to plasma concentration at time t of what is administered at time s, only the difference $t - s$ matters. More precisely, this assumption implies that $G(t, s) = G(t - s)$ where $G(t)$ is the response curve to a unit bolus dose given at time 0.

This is computable as a difference of two observable quantities:

$$\mathrm{MAT} = \mathrm{MRT}_{app} - \mathrm{MRT}_{iv}.$$

Note that the relation

$$I(C) = DI(G),$$

for a linear PK system shows that if we study different doses, then $I(C)$ should be proportional to absorbed dose, not the given dose. This distinction is important when the dose is given to an extravascular site, like the intestines. Different doses may have different absolute bioavailabilities, and then a plot of $I(C)$ versus given dose is not a straight line through the origin. There are different reasons why bioavailability may differ between doses. A simple one is that if much drug is given there may not be time to absorb it all before the drug leaves the site of absorption.

2.3.2 Intravascular infusion

We have already noted that the bolus dose we have assumed for much of the discussion above is an abstract concept. Intravascular doses are given as infusions in a controlled way, so that we know the exact flow of drug into plasma at each time. This means that the function $a(t)$ is completely known.

In its simplest form we give a fixed amount per time unit, R, for a given time τ, so that the absorption rate is given by $a(t) = R \cdot I_{[0,\tau]}(t)$. (The term absorption is often reserved for drug transfer from a site into the blood stream, but we do not make that distinction.) Thus the dose we give is obtained from $D = R\tau$, and we see that

$$\mathrm{MAT} = \frac{\int_0^\tau s\,ds}{\int_0^\tau ds} = \frac{\tau}{2}.$$

We keep the notation MAT, though it might be more proper to call this the Mean Infusion Time, denoted MIT.

By measuring the resulting plasma concentration $C(t)$, we obtain $G(t)$ by solving the equation

$$C(t) = (a * G)(t) = R \int_0^t G(t-s) I_{[0,\tau]}(s)\,ds.$$

Let a primitive function to $G(t)$ be defined by

$$G_*(t) = \int_0^t G(s)\,ds.$$

Then, if $t < \tau$

$$C(t) = R \int_0^t G(t-s)\,ds = RG_*(t), \tag{2.13}$$

whereas if $t > \tau$

$$C(t) = R \int_0^\tau G(t-s)\,ds = R(G_*(t) - G_*(t-\tau)). \tag{2.14}$$

This determines $G_*(t)$, and therefore its derivative $G(t)$.

As an example, let $G(t) = Ae^{-\lambda t}$. Then $G_*(t) = (A/\lambda)(1 - e^{-\lambda t})$, and for $t > \tau$ we have

$$C(t) = \frac{RA}{\lambda}((1 - e^{-\lambda t}) - (1 - e^{-\lambda(t-\tau)})) = \frac{RA(e^{\lambda \tau} - 1)}{\lambda} e^{-\lambda t}.$$

One of the consequences of replacing a bolus dose with an infusion is that we lose the direct access to V_c, since now $C(0) = 0$. But we can use the computation above to obtain an estimate. Thus, if we approximate $C(t)$ with a mono-exponential for a short time after the end of infusion, $C(t) \approx Be^{-\lambda t}$, we can deduce that for the time interval in question

$$G(t) \approx \frac{B\lambda}{R(e^{\lambda \tau} - 1)} e^{-\lambda t}.$$

If this is a good approximation also for small t, for instance, if τ is small, it follows that

$$V_c = \frac{1}{G(0)} = \frac{D(e^{\lambda \tau} - 1)}{B\lambda \tau}, \tag{2.15}$$

which gives us a way to estimate the volume of the central compartment in the case of a non-bolus infusion.

Before we leave the case of intravascular infusion, let us note the following. In order to obtain $G(t)$ we need to measure the plasma concentration $C_\tau(t)$ after intravenous infusion for some time τ. We can then obtain $G(t)$ from the equation

$$C_\tau(t) = R(I_{[0,\tau]} * G)(t).$$

We do not need to solve this explicitly to be able to solve equation 2.12 for the absorption rate $a(t)$. Instead we can solve the equation

$$C(t) = (a_\tau * C_\tau)(t),$$

in which we have both $C(t)$ and $C_\tau(t)$ and then reconstruct $a(t)$ from $a_\tau(t)$ by

$$a(t) = R(a_\tau * I_{[0,\tau]})(t) = R \int_{t-\tau}^{t} a_\tau(s)\,ds, \quad t > \tau.$$

To see this, just insert the expressions:

$$(a * G)(t) = C(t) = (a_\tau * C_\tau)(t) = (a_\tau * RI_{[0,\tau]} * G)(t).$$

2.3.3 Extravascular drug administration

The most common extravascular site of administration is the gastrointesti-nal (GI) tract, which is the site of absorption when the drug is given as a solution or a tablet. Other extravascular administration sites include in-tramuscular and subcutaneous injections. Some drugs are administered by inhalation through the lungs. This includes not only narcotic gases, but also some treatments for respiratory diseases like asthma. Extravascular admin-istration of a drug is from a pharmacokinetics point of view a more complex process than intravascular administration, especially for drugs taken up from the GI tract. If you swallow a tablet, this first has to dissolve, so that the sub-stance gets into solution in the intestinal juice before the process of actually absorbing the substance through the gastrointestinal wall can start. All drug may not be dissolved from the dosage form, to become absorbed, leading to incomplete absorption from the intestines.

Another complication is that the only thing we can measure is what is in plasma. Even if a drug is completely absorbed from the intestines it may be metabolized (and therefore eliminated) both in the walls of the intestines, and, more importantly perhaps, in the liver. Anatomically, a drug molecule that appears in the vein we sample from needs to have passed through both the intestine walls and the liver. This is called the *first pass effect*, and explains why the dose we see in plasma may be lower than the dose primarily absorbed.

In all this means that

1. we do not actually know the dose that enters the blood stream, and

2. the details on how it enters cannot be modelled very accurately.

So we take an altogether empirical approach to absorption. We use a probabilistic description: imagine a dose D *given*, which consists of a very large number of drug molecules. Let $F(t)$ be the fraction of dose given that has presented itself in the blood stream at time t. The rate at which it enters plasma is then given by

$$a(t) = DF'(t) = FDf(t),$$

where the bioavailability parameter F is $F(\infty) =$ total fraction of dose given that is absorbed (i.e., seen in plasma) and $f(t) = F'(t)/F(\infty)$. So $f(t)$ is a probability density function which describes time to being absorbed for a molecule that actually is absorbed. The expected value of this is the Mean Absorption Time, MAT.

In principle any distribution on positive numbers can serve as an absorption distribution, the simplest being the exponential distribution for which

$$f(t) = k_a e^{-k_a t}.$$

This is called a first order absorption process with absorption rate k_a. The MAT for this distribution is $1/k_a$. We can visualize this case as follows. Let $D(t)$ be the amount of drug not absorbed at time t. If this dissolves with a constant rate:

$$D'(t) = -k_a D(t), \quad D(0) = D,$$

and a fraction F of what is dissolved makes it the whole way to be presented in the blood stream we have $a(t) = -FD'(t) = FDk_a e^{-k_a t}$.

For future use we compute $C(t)$ for a first order absorption process when $G(t) = e^{-\lambda t}$:

$$C(t) = (FDk_a e^{-k_a t} * e^{-\lambda t})(t) = \frac{FDk_a}{k_a - \lambda}(e^{-\lambda t} - e^{-k_a t}).$$

The exponential distribution is by far the one most used in pharmacokinetics to describe absorption. This is to a large extent due to its good computational relation to the polyexponential function description of bolus doses, as indicated by the computation above. It has its short-comings: if a tablet is given that is dissolved and absorbed only in the small intestines, it does take some time until absorption starts, since the drug first has to go through the stomach which therefore has to be emptied before absorption commences. This is usually handled by the introduction of a lag-time, t_{lag}, which is meant to describe the time it takes from swallowing to emptying of the ventricle, thus setting the clock for absorption. Practically this means that, for a first order absorption,

$$a(t) = 0, t < t_{lag}, \quad a(t) = FDk_a e^{-k_a(t-t_{lag})}, t > t_{lag}.$$

For such an absorption process we have that

$$\text{MAT} = t_{lag} + \frac{1}{k_a}.$$

For non-bolus single dose administration there are two new basic PK parameters which are always presented

C_{max}: which is the maximal concentration, and

t_{max}: which is time at which this peak concentration occurs.

For an intravenous infusion with a constant rate, it is clear that $t_{max} = \tau =$ end of infusion time. The peak concentration in turn can be expressed in terms of the infusion rate R and the unit dose bolus response $G(t)$ as

$$C_{max} = R \int_0^\tau G(t)\, dt.$$

In the extravascular case, differentiating the formula $C(t) = (a * G)(t)$ we get

$$C'(t) = G(t)a(0) + (G * a')(t).$$

For a first order absorbing process for which $a'(t) = -k_a a(t)$, we have that the second term becomes $k_a(G * a)(t) = -k_a C(t)$ and the equation becomes

$$C'(t) = G(t)k_a FD - k_a C(t).$$

From this we can obtain estimates for k_a if we know the fraction F absorbed: integrate over the interval (t_1, t_2) to obtain

$$k_a = \frac{C(t_2) - C(t_1)}{\int_{t_1}^{t_2} (FDG(s) - C(s))\, ds}. \tag{2.16}$$

We can do this over different intervals, possibly obtaining different rates, from which an approximative absorption profile can be obtained.

Still under the assumption of a first order absorption process, and no lagtime, we can also note that the condition for t_{max} is that at this point we have

$$C'(t) = k_a(FDG(t) - C(t)) = 0,$$

so the ratio

$$\frac{C(t_{max})}{G(t_{max})} = FD = \frac{\int_0^\infty C(t)\, dt}{\int_0^\infty G(t)\, dt}$$

equals the amount absorbed. This formula, $C_{max} = FDG(t_{max})$, shows that the later we have t_{max}, the smaller will C_{max} be. For the case $G(t) = e^{-\lambda t}$ this criteria becomes

$$\frac{FDk_a}{k_a - \lambda}(e^{-\lambda t} - e^{-k_a t}) = FDe^{-\lambda t} \quad \Longleftrightarrow \quad t_{max} = \frac{1}{k_a - \lambda}\ln\left(\frac{k_a}{\lambda}\right).$$

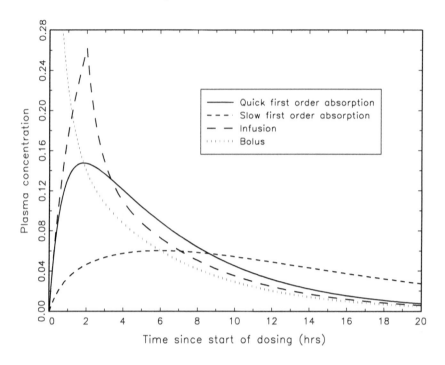

FIGURE 2.2: Plasma profiles after different types of single dose administrations. The dose absorbed is the same for all curves.

An illustration is given in Figure 2.2 of the effect of an absorption process, as opposed to a prompt bolus. Note that according to the theory above the area (to infinity) under all these curves is the same. Also note the relationship between t_{max} and C_{max}: the later the former, the smaller the latter. In fact, for this particular case t_{max} occurs when the plasma curve intersects the bolus-curve, because we have $F = 1$.

If the absorption rate k_a is small enough, it may even be smaller than the slowest elimination rate obtained after a bolus administration. Then the terminal phase seen in plasma after this administration is determined by the absorption rate, so that $\lambda_{el} = k_a$. This phenomenon is called a "flip-flop" phenomena.

2.4 Multiple dosing

As in the previous section, we will in this section assume a linear PK system. That means in particular that conclusions drawn in this section can be used as tests for the linearity of a pharmacokinetics system.

We will consider multiple dosing of the same drug. In real life in particular the absorption after GI administrations can be very variable from time to time. However, mathematically we assume that all doses given produce the same individual plasma concentrations $C(t)$. So, we assume that we take doses at times

$$0 = \tau_0 < \tau_1 < \ldots \tau_n,$$

and that each dose contributes the same plasma concentration $C(t)$ to the total concentration. For time $t > \tau_n$ we then have that the accumulated plasma concentration is

$$\sum_{i=0}^{n} C(t - \tau_i),$$

since dose i taken at time τ_i contributes the concentration $C(t - \tau_i)$ to the total concentration at time t. This shows us how to construct the total plasma concentration after each new dose. An illustration is shown in Figure 2.3.

Many drugs have a therapeutic window within which we want our plasma concentrations to lie over a dosing interval. Lower concentrations than those of the lower limit of this window are perceived to be ineffective, whereas higher concentrations than those of the upper limit may be associated with potentially dangerous side-effects. If we have a drug with a therapeutic window, we want to adjust dosage interval and dosage formulation (i.e., modifying the uptake rate function $a(t)$) so that the plasma concentration curve stays within the therapeutic window, like that in Figure 2.3.

Now we start the clock after the nth dose instead of after the first dose. This means that we take as time not t but $t - \tau_n$. With this re-timing we find that the concentration after the nth dose is given by

$$C_n(t) = \sum_{i=0}^{n} C(t + \tau_n - \tau_i).$$

Also assume that all dosing intervals have the same length, so that $\tau_{i+1} - \tau_i = \tau$ for all i. Since

$$\tau_n - \tau_i = (\tau_n - \tau_{n-1}) + \ldots + (\tau_{i+1} - \tau_i) = (n - i)\tau$$

we see that we have

$$C_n(t) = \sum_{i=0}^{n} C(t + i\tau) \to C_{ss}(t) \text{ as } t \to \infty.$$

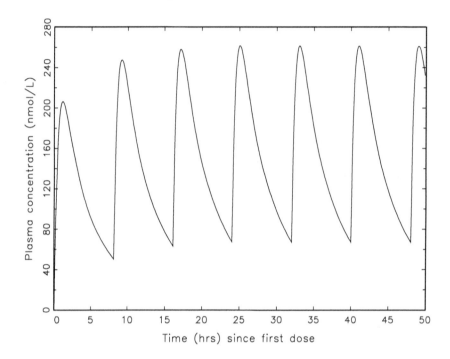

FIGURE 2.3: Plasma concentration profile when multiple, identical doses are given every 8th hour

The limiting concentration here is called the *concentration in steady state* though it is not the same kind of steady state we have with a continuous infusion – it is steady state with respect to dosing.

What, then, characterizes $C_{ss}(t)$? Our notation means that we follow $C_{ss}(t)$ from the last dose in steady state, and at time t we have a contribution to $C_{ss}(t)$ both from the last dose given and from all the previous ones. The latter contribution is $C_{ss}(t + \tau)$, so we get the relation

$$C_{ss}(t) = C(t) + C_{ss}(t + \tau). \qquad (2.17)$$

This formula is a summary of our assumptions, and it has two immediate consequences:

1. The integral over a period in steady state equals the total integral after a single dose:

$$\int_0^\tau C_{ss}(t)\, dt = \int_0^\infty C(t)\, dt.$$

In fact, $I(C)$ equals

$$\int_0^\infty C_{ss}(t)\, dt - \int_0^\infty C_{ss}(t + \tau)\, dt = \int_0^\infty C_{ss}(t)\, dt - \int_\tau^\infty C_{ss}(t)\, dt.$$

2. The MRT_{app} (i.e., $E(C)/I(C)$) from a single dose can be computed from steady state data as

$$\mathrm{MRT}_{app} = \frac{\int_0^\tau tC_{ss}(t)dt + \tau \int_\tau^\infty C_{ss}(t)dt}{\int_0^\tau C_{ss}(t)dt}.$$

This follows from the observation

$$\int_0^\infty tC(t)\, dt = \int_0^\infty tC_{ss}(t)\, dt - \int_\tau^\infty (t-\tau)C_{ss}(t)\, dt$$

and what we have already shown.

There are two new PK parameters of interest in multiple dosing situations:

C_{min}: which is the minimal concentration and

t_{min}: which is the time point of occurrence of the minimal concentration.

In most cases this refers to the trough concentrations, i.e., the concentration just before the next dose $(C_{ss}(\tau))$, so that $t_{min} = \tau$. Another descriptor of interest for steady state is the accumulation ratio

$$R_{ac}(t) = \frac{C_{ss}(t)}{C(t)} = 1 + \frac{C_{ss}(t+\tau)}{C(t)}, \quad 0 \le t \le \tau.$$

As such it is a function of time, and in order to describe accumulation by only one number, we may use its value at $t = \tau$ or, alternatively, we may use the area ratio

$$R_{ac} = \frac{\int_0^\tau C_{ss}(t)\, dt}{\int_0^\tau C(t)\, dt},$$

which is the ratio of the mean concentrations over the dosing interval. Note that this is a number we can predict from single dose data, by computing instead the ratio

$$R_{pac} = \frac{\int_0^\infty C(t)\, dt}{\int_0^\tau C(t)\, dt}.$$

In order to see how accumulation changes the shape of the plasma concentration curve, as compared to the first dose, first consider the simple monoexponential $C(t) = e^{-\lambda t}$. Then

$$C_{ss}(t) = \sum_{i=0}^\infty e^{-\lambda(t+i\tau)} = e^{-\lambda t}\sum_{i=0}^\infty (e^{-\lambda\tau})^i = \frac{e^{-\lambda t}}{1 - e^{-\lambda\tau}},$$

which shows that in this case

$$R_{ac}(t) = \frac{1}{1 - e^{-\lambda\tau}},$$

independent of t. The same result is obtained if we divide the areas.

This computation immediately extends to polyexponentials:

$$C(t) = \sum_{i=1}^{K} A_i e^{-\lambda_i t} \implies C_{ss}(t) = \sum_{i=1}^{K} \frac{A_i}{1 - e^{-\lambda_i \tau}} e^{-\lambda_i t}. \tag{2.18}$$

Since $1 - e^{-\lambda_i \tau}$ is the smallest and its reciprocal the largest for the smallest λ_i we see that the coefficients for slow phases increase most, with the effect of the terminal elimination rate being largest. The next example will illustrate this change of the profile of the plasma concentration curve.

Example 2.2

As an example, consider the drug of Example 2.1 with a bolus dose of 10 mg given every eighth hour. Then the single dose and steady state curves are

$$C(t) = 0.38e^{-1.65t} + 0.18e^{-0.182t}, \quad C_{ss}(t) = 0.38e^{-1.65t} + 0.23e^{-0.182t}.$$

We see that the effect on the first coefficient is very small whereas the second is increased by 30%.

An illustration of this is given in Figure 2.4, where the single dose and steady state curves are shown together. We see that at dosing time the difference (a ratio since the scale is logarithmic) is small, but it increases with time. This is because the main effect is on the second phase, and effects are seen as this phase starts to contribute to the overall concentration. We also find a plot of the function $R_{ac}(t)$, which starts at approximately a 10% increase and levels off at 30%. For comparison, the eight hour area ratio is $R_{ac} = 1.23$.

Not surprisingly most of the accumulation occurs after one dose. In fact, the plasma curve after the nth dose is given by

$$C_n(t) = \sum_{i=1}^{K} A_i \frac{1 - e^{-n\lambda_i \tau}}{1 - e^{-\lambda_i \tau}} e^{-\lambda_i t},$$

which shows, with our parameter values, that the second coefficient has risen from 0.18 to 0.22 already for the second dose. So, for practical purposes, with these elimination rates we are in steady state already after the second, or possibly the third (depending on your standards) dose in this case. □

If the absorption process is not complete within a dosing interval, also this process will have effects on the shape of the plasma concentration curve in steady state. How this influences peak concentration and the time for it is left to the interested reader.

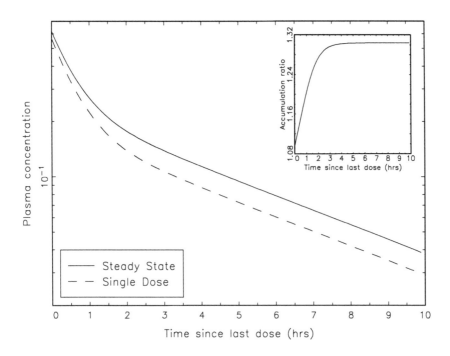

FIGURE 2.4: The plasma profile after single dose and in steady state after last dose, for bolus dose administrations

2.5 One compartment drugs with capacity limited elimination

In this section we will have a closer look at one-compartmental drugs, i.e., drugs that do not have a distribution phase. For such drugs there is only one volume, V, and equation 2.2 takes the form

$$VC'(t) = a(t) - CL(t)C(t).$$

If, in addition, clearance is constant, and we give a bolus dose D, we get

$$C(t) = \frac{D}{V}e^{-CLt/V},$$

and for a general administration we have the formula

$$C(t) = V^{-1}\int_0^t e^{-CL(t-s)/V}a(s)\,ds.$$

A quick computations shows that in this case the mean residence time is

$$\text{MRT} = \frac{V}{CL}.$$

More interesting is the case of capacity limited elimination. We may, e.g., assume that our drug is eliminated in the liver by a metabolic pathway for which there is a limited supply of enzymes. We can model this by assuming that there are constants v_m, K_m such that

$$CL(t) = \frac{v_m}{K_m + C(t)}.$$

In fact, we can allow the drug to be eliminated both by renal excretion and by metabolism, and therefore assume that we have the basic model equation

$$VC'(t) = a(t) - (CL_R + \frac{v_m}{K_m + C(t)})C(t). \qquad (2.19)$$

We now consider what happens when we give a bolus dose D. When the dose is low, and concentrations small compared to K_m, we have almost a straight line, since then clearance is essentially constant. When we increase the dose we get two "phases", of which the faster phase is the last one. During the first phase, when concentration is large compared to K_m, we have a constant amount of drug eliminated per time unit, given by v_m. Such elimination is called zero order elimination in pharmacokinetics. As the concentration decreases, this eventually turns into a first order elimination with rate $CL_{tot} = CL_R + v_m/K_m$ for very small concentrations. In particular this means that the terminal elimination rate is

$$k_{el} = \frac{CL_{tot}}{V}.$$

One drug for which this applies is alcohol. Plasma concentrations after bolus administration of different volumes of 40% v/v whisky are shown in Figure 2.5. Alcohol is metabolized in the liver, by enzymes of limited capacity. This metabolism can at least approximately be described by the function in equation 2.19 with no renal clearance and with $v_m = 10$ g/h and $K_m = 100$ mg/L. The doses given in Figure 2.5 are a tenth of a typical drink, one drink and five drinks. The pharmacological effects appear at a concentration of about 200 mg/L, which is the dashed line in Figure 2.5. We see that the first curve shows no non-linearity, but that with increasing doses non-linearity becomes more pronounced. Note that the effect duration increases more than proportionally to the number of drinks taken.

We now want to derive formulas for the basic PK parameters in the case of a one-compartmental drug with capacity-limited elimination. For this we need to compute two key integrals, and how this can be done is shown in

---

Box 2.2 Deriving the AUC and MRT parameters for the saturated one-compartmental model for a bolus dose

---

In order to study a system like this, it is best first to make it non-dimensional. Introducing

$$\tau = \frac{v_m}{K_m V}, \quad s = \tau t, \quad f = \frac{K_m CL_R}{v_m}, \quad y(s) = C(t)/K_m, \quad y_0 = D/V K_m,$$

we find the following differential equation

$$y'(s) = -(f + \frac{1}{1 + y(s)})y(s), \quad y(0) = y_0$$

for $y(s)$. We can rearrange and integrate this to

$$\int_0^\infty y(s)ds = -\frac{1}{1+f} \int_0^\infty \frac{1 + y(s)}{1 + gy(s)} y'(s)ds = \frac{1}{f}(y_0 - \frac{1}{f}\ln(1 + gy_0))$$

with $g = f/(1 + f)$. A similar argument shows that with

$$\int_0^\infty s(1 + \frac{1}{1 + y(s)})y(s)ds = -\int_0^\infty sy'(s)ds = \int_0^\infty y(s)ds.$$

In the special case $g = f = 0$ we get

$$\int_0^\infty y(s)^k ds = -\int_0^\infty (1 + y(s))y(s)^{k-1}y'(s)ds = \frac{y_0^k}{k} + \frac{y_0^{k+1}}{k+1}$$

and also that

$$\int_0^\infty sy(s)ds = -\int_0^\infty (1 + y(s))sy'(s)ds = \int_0^\infty (y(s) + y(s)^2/2)ds$$

so that

$$\frac{\int_0^\infty sy(s)ds}{\int_0^\infty y(s)ds} = 1 + \frac{\int_0^\infty y(s)^2 ds}{2\int_0^\infty y(s)ds} = 1 + \frac{y_0^2/2 + y_0^3/3}{2y_0 + y_0^2} = 1 + \frac{1}{6}\frac{3y_0 + 2y_0^2}{2 + y_0}.$$

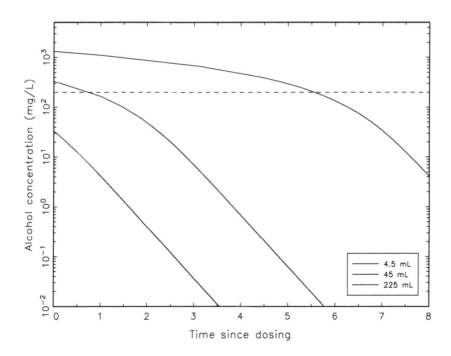

FIGURE 2.5: Plasma concentrations after different bolus doses of 40% v/v
              whiskey

Box 2.2. Back-substituting in the formulas derived there first gives a total
area

$$\int_0^\infty C(t)\,dt = \frac{D}{CL_R} - \frac{V v_m}{CL_R^2} \ln(1 + \frac{D}{VK_m}\frac{CL_R}{CL_{tot}}).$$

If we let $CL_R \to 0$, we find that if there is only metabolic clearance the
integral is a quadratic function of dose and not a linear one as in the case of
linear kinetics:

$$\int_0^\infty C(t)\,dt = \frac{D}{CL_{tot}}(1 + \frac{D}{2VK_m}).$$

So the area is not proportional to D, it is a quadratic function of D, and the
average clearance is dose dependent:

$$CL_{av} = \frac{D}{\int_0^\infty C(t)\,dt} = \frac{v_m}{K_m + D/2V}.$$

Returning to the general case with renal clearance, if we integrate Equation 2.19 after pre-multiplication with t, we see that

$$\int_0^\infty tCL(t)C(t)dt = V\int_0^\infty C(t)dt$$

so the mean residence time is given by

$$\text{MRT} = \frac{V}{CL_R} - \frac{V^2 v_m}{DCL_R^2} \ln(1 + \frac{D}{VK_m}\frac{CL_R}{CL_{tot}}),$$

which is an increasing function of D. When we only have metabolic clearance it is a straight line:

$$\text{MRT} = \frac{VK_m}{v_m} + \frac{D}{2v_m}.$$

The apparent MRT is slightly more involved (see Box 2.2):

$$\text{MRT}_{app} = \frac{VK_m}{v_m} + \frac{D}{4v_m}\frac{1 + 2D/3VK_m}{1 + D/2VK_m} \approx \frac{VK_m}{v_m} + \frac{D}{4v_m}$$

when $C(0) = D/V$ is small, but $\approx VK_m/v_m + D/3v_m$ when $C(0)$ is large. Compared to the true MRT the apparent MRT increases first with only half the rate per unit dose increase.

This has consequences for the estimate of volumes. The true V_{ss}, defined as $CL_{av}\text{MRT}$, is found from the formulas above to be V, as it should be. However, applying NCA techniques to this data we obtain

$$V_{ss} = CL_{av}\text{MRT}_{app} = V - \frac{D}{4K_m}\frac{1 + D/3VK_m}{(1 + D/2VK_m)^2}.$$

When $C(0)$ is small this is approximately equal to V, but when $C(0)$ is large it is approximately $2V/3$, and we will always underestimate the true volume using V_{ss} as our estimate. For the volume of distribution we have

$$V_d = \frac{CL_{av}}{v_m/VK_m} = \frac{V}{1 + D/2VK_m},$$

so it is also underestimated.

The lesson learned from this is that with non-linearity present (at least on clearance) our non-compartmental standard PK parameters may not be very good estimates of what they are supposed to estimate. Both the volume and the mean residence time are typically underestimated.

To detect deviation from linearity, we plot $I(C)$, or AUC in standard PK terminology, versus dose. We know that for a linear PK system we should have a direct proportionality. If we therefore give increasing doses and find that $I(C)$ as a function of dose is not proportional to dose, we do not have a linear system. If $I(C)$ increases faster than proportional to dose, we may have capacity limited elimination.

2.6 Chapter epilogue: A recirculation model

In the discussion above we have considered the body to be like a container filled with water which we enter drug into and remove drug from. We sample from a special part of the container (the blood) but we do not really concern ourselves with what happens within the container. Instead we produce an empirical, non-physiological description of it as a container with a fixed concentration and a varying volume. This results in pharmacokinetics concepts and parameters that are useful for comparing different drugs. In this section we will look at an alternative modelling approach that gives some further insight into the meaning of these PK parameters.

What our standard model does not account for is the circulatory system present in all vertebrates. In the alternative approach we instead focus on the fact that when we sample we look into the circulatory system at one particular point; denote it P. We let $C(t)$ be drug blood concentration at time t at this point, and let the blood flow at that point be denoted Q (if we measure plasma concentrations, this is plasma flow). Then $QC(t)$ is the amount of drug passing the point P at time t per time unit. A good point to take measurements at is a point physiologically equivalent to the right atrium in which case the blood flow is the cardiac output.

A drug molecule that passes at time t may either be there for the first time or have passed the point at some previous time. A molecule that passes P at a particular time can either return to this point after some time, the circulation time, or be eliminated during this circulation so that it does not return. Let E denote the whole body extraction ratio, i.e., the fraction of drug molecules that start its circulation and is eliminated from the system during that circulation (we assume linearity so that this is not time dependent). The one-pass circulation function $H(t)$ is defined as the fraction of molecules that passed the point P at time 0 that return to P for the first time at the particular time t. Then

$$\int_0^\infty H(t)\,dt = 1 - E,$$

since a drug that was not eliminated during its circulation must reappear.

The fundamental mass-balance equation for this modelling approach will now be

$$QC(t) = a(t) + Q(H * C)(t), \tag{2.20}$$

where $a(t)$ is the flow of drug that appears for the first time at the point P at time t.

Integration of equation 2.20 gives us $QI(C) = I(a) + QI(H)I(C)$, and since $I(a) = D$ is the dose given, we find that $I(C) = D/Q(1 - I(H)) = D/QE$.

Thus the extraction ratio is given by

$$E = \frac{D}{Q \int_0^\infty C(t)\, dt},$$

and we see that QE is the clearance CL_{av}. Note that both Q and $H(t)$ depend on where in the circulatory system we sample, but QE does not.

Applying the operator $E(.)$ to Equation 2.20 gives us, after some rearrangement, that

$$\frac{E(C)}{I(C)} = \frac{E(a)}{D} + \frac{E(H)}{1 - I(H)}.$$

We define the mean circulation time t_{circ} by

$$t_{circ} = \frac{E(H)}{I(H)} = \frac{\int_0^\infty t H(t)\, dt}{\int_0^\infty H(t)\, dt},$$

and we find that we have the following expression for the apparent mean residence time

$$\mathrm{MRT}_{app} = \mathrm{MAT} + \frac{1 - E}{E} t_{circ}.$$

The coefficient $(1 - E)/E$ is therefore the number of circulations a molecule on average make before being eliminated.

The reasoning in this section will reappear in Chapter 4, where functions corresponding to the one-pass circulation function $H(t)$ will be defined for individual organs and then assembled into a full organism. We will also discuss the recirculation model of this section further in Chapter 5.

Chapter 3

Numerical methods for PK parameter estimation

3.1 Introduction

In this chapter we will address how we can numerically compute from observed data the parameters and other quantities, discussed in the previous chapter. In real life we do not get plasma concentration data as polyexponential functions. Instead we determine a series of time points (relative to dosing) at which blood samples are taken and plasma concentrations are measured. The quality of those data, as estimates of the true plasma concentration profile, depends on our choice of time points. An inappropriate choice may make us miss the peak concentration or we may not have sampled long enough to obtain a good estimate of the terminal elimination rate.

But we have to work with what we have and in this chapter we will look into numerical aspects of the computation of the PK parameters. As already noted, most PK parameters depend on a few integrals, and estimating those in turn in general requires an estimate of the terminal elimination rate. This is because most integrals are over $[0, \infty)$, but we cannot sample the whole interval. To remedy that, we use a mono-exponential approximation after the last true measurement point, based on the concentration at that point and the terminal elimination rate.

One further comment before we begin the discussion on numerical methods. Very small plasma concentrations cannot be measured. Therefore each assay method has a certain threshold, called the Limit Of Quantification (LOQ) below which no concentration can be measured. Instead we only know that the concentration is less than LOQ. This means that even though such concentrations are missing, they represent informative missing since we know that they are missing because they are lower than a particular value, LOQ. This fact poses some problems which will soon be discussed.

3.2   Estimating the terminal elimination rate

The obvious way to estimate the terminal elimination rate is to plot $\ln C(t)$ versus t, and to fit a straight line using linear regression to the later parts of the curve, choosing a portion which is reasonably close to a straight line.

The main problem is that we may not be able to identify the terminal elimination rate correctly. We may not have followed the plasma curve for a sufficiently long period, or our assay method is not sensitive enough to allow the quantification of slow phases at low concentrations. From a technical perspective these two cases amount to the same problem.

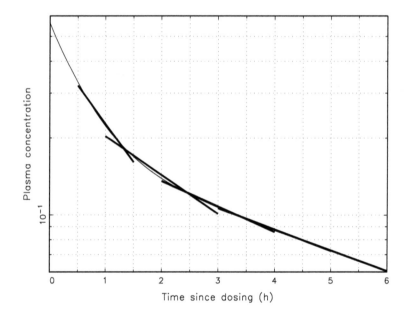

FIGURE 3.1: Drawing terminal elimination lines based on different LOQ

In Figure 3.1 we illustrate the problems with incomplete assessment of the terminal phase. We have assumed that we follow the curve for different lengths of time, and for each such time period, we use the last 2 hours to estimate the terminal elimination rate, illustrated as the straight lines in the graph. We see that a shorter observation period (or less sensitive assay methods) leads to underestimation of the terminal half-life: for the first line it is only one hour, for the third it is three hours and for the last it is close to the correct 3.76 hours. The increase is because we catch up with the second, and in this case last, phase of the curve as the assay improves (LOQ becomes smaller).

But this is under the assumption that we actually get a nice and smooth curve from the data. In reality there is some noise in data, partly due to assay precision, partly to physiological effects on the individual during the course of the experiment. Also, we only get a relatively small number of data points since getting many would deplete the subject under investigation of his blood. One problem is to find an algorithm that identifies an appropriate range over which the linear regression is to be done. One such algorithm, which has long served this author well, but always needs to be supplemented by a sanity check, goes as follows:

1. Use the last three points to make a linear regression on and compute the R^2 to this linear regression.

2. Successively add earlier time points and make the linear regression on these data until the R^2 decreases (i.e., degree of explanation decreases).

3. When a point for which a R^2 decrease is encountered, remove that point and add the preceding one. Repeat the analysis. If R^2 still decreases, the process is stopped and the data are included in the linear regression up to the first decrease in R^2. If however R^2 increases, we consider the removed point an outlier and continue the process with that individual point removed.

This is not a fool-proof method but it usually represents a good starting point. However, sometimes one needs to use only the last two points in the estimate of the terminal slope, which this method does not allow for (no R^2 can be computed in that case). Data must therefore always be inspected in order to allow for manual modification of the time interval over which the regression should be made.

Often the terminal elimination rate is based only on a small number of low concentrations. One could supplement the method above with a re-estimation step, in which information is borrowed between individuals. Three points may lie more or less on a straight line, but if the first is, by chance, slightly too low and the last is slightly too high, we may get a far too long terminal half-life estimate. It may then be useful to estimate conditional on what other estimates are. The way this can be done is using a linear mixed effects model as follows. Select all data points that regression was based on in the previous step and estimate parameters in the mixed effects model $\ln C = a - bt$, with both parameters a and b random. Then use the so-called empirical Bayes estimates of individual effects as your new individual parameter estimates. Intuitively this method should produce more reliable estimates for data where the fit to the line is poor, but it does not seem to have been discussed in the literature. We will not use this updating method in our example in Section 3.6.2.

A completely different approach to the estimation of the terminal elimination rate is to compute the derivatives $C'(t)$ numerically at each point, and then plot the points $(C(t), C'(t))$. Close to $(0,0)$ in this graph one should have a relation $C'(t) = -k_{el}C(t)$, from which we can estimate k_{el}. However, this method does not seem to have any numerical advantages over the simple linear regression method discussed above.

One final note on the terminal elimination rate. As pointed out, assay sensitivity or a limited observation time can hide a longer terminal elimination phase. One way to get a hint of a hidden longer phase can be obtained from the accumulation ratio at the trough value, if multiple dosing data are available. If we assume that only the terminal elimination phase contributes to this, we would have

$$R_{ac}(\tau) = \frac{1}{1 - e^{-\lambda_{el}\tau}}, \tag{3.1}$$

where τ is the dosing interval, from which we can estimate λ_{el}.

3.3   Integral estimation

In order to compute the pharmacokinetics parameters, we need to compute a number of integrals, since the basic PK parameters are based on the two integrals

$$I(C) = \int_0^\infty C(t)\, dt, \qquad E(C) = \int_0^\infty tC(t)\, dt.$$

We have illustrated the computations of PK parameters so far, assuming that we have polyexponential functions for $C(t)$, which are easily integrated. In real life we have a sequence $(t_i, C_i), i = 0, \ldots, n$, (with $t_0 = 0$) of data points from which we want to estimate the integrals. The problem is divided into two parts: to compute the integral over the range of observation $[0, t_n]$ and to compute the extrapolated area over $[t_n, \infty)$.

The extrapolated area is computed by finding an estimate of a terminal elimination rate λ, either from the data at hand or from other data (as from an intravenous administration). Then we assume that

$$C(t) = C_n e^{-\lambda(t - t_n)}, \quad t > t_n,$$

where C_n is the concentration measured at t_n, which is the last one that is above LOQ. From this we compute

$$\int_{t_n}^\infty C(t)\, dt = C_n \int_0^\infty e^{-\lambda s}\, ds = \frac{C_n}{\lambda},$$

$$\int_{t_n}^\infty tC(t)\, dt = C_n \int_0^\infty (s + t_n)e^{-\lambda s}\, ds = C_n\left(\frac{1}{\lambda^2} + \frac{t_n}{\lambda}\right).$$

In order to compute the integral over $[0, t_n]$ we can choose between different approaches. The simplest is to pretend that we have a piecewise linear function. This means that we can use the trapeze formula

$$\int_0^{t_n} C(t)\, dt = \sum_{i=1}^{n} \frac{C_i + C_{i-1}}{2}(t_i - t_{i-1}).$$

With this method we assume that the integrand ($C(t)$ or $tC(t)$) is piecewise linear; so in order to integrate $tC(t)$ we just replace C_i with $t_i C_i$.

An alternative method is to approximate the integrand with quadratics, defined by each triplet of points, and integrate that. This is Simpson's formula

$$\int_0^{t_n} C(t)\, dt = \sum_{i=1}^{n} \left(\frac{C_{i-1} + 4C_i + C_{i+1}}{6}(t_{i+1} - t_{i-1}) \right) +$$

$$\sum_{i=1}^{n} \left(\frac{C_{i-1} + C_{i+1}}{3}(t_{i+1} + t_{i-1} - 2t_i) \right).$$

The first sum is what appears in the standard Simpson formula for equidistant points; the second sum is called Brun's modification for non-equidistant points. Again, integrating $tC(t)$ we just replace C_i with $t_i C_i$.

In pharmacokinetics there is one more method, which probably is the most popular one. It is based on the observation of the fundamental role exponential functions play in making up plasma concentration curves, especially after bolus dosing. It is called the log-trapeze method and assumes that within the interval $[t_i, t_{i+1}]$ the form of $C(t)$ is $Ae^{\lambda t}$. Parameters A and λ are determined from

$$Ae^{\lambda t_i} = C_i, \quad Ae^{\lambda t_{i+1}} = C_{i+1},$$

which we solve as

$$\lambda = \frac{\ln(C_{i+1}/C_i)}{t_{i+1} - t_i}, \quad A = C_i e^{-\lambda t_i}.$$

It then follows that

$$\int_{t_i}^{t_{i+1}} C(t)\, dt = \frac{A}{\lambda}(e^{\lambda t_{i+1}} - e^{\lambda t_i}) = \frac{C_{i+1} - C_i}{\ln(C_{i+1}/C_i)}(t_{i+1} - t_i),$$

so the log-trapeze formula is

$$\int_0^{t_n} C(t)\, dt = \sum_{i=1}^{n} \frac{C_{i+1} - C_i}{\ln(C_{i+1}/C_i)}(t_{i+1} - t_i).$$

However, if we want to integrate $tC(t)$ here, we should be a bit cautious. The assumption is that the plasma concentration is a piecewise exponential, so $tC(t)$ is not. Instead we need to compute

$$\int_{t_i}^{t_{i+1}} tAe^{\lambda t}\, dt = \frac{t_{i+1} - t_i}{\ln(C_{i+1}/C_i)} \left((t_{i+1}C_{i+1} - t_i C_i) - (C_{i+1} - C_i)\frac{t_{i+1} - t_i}{\ln(C_{i+1}/C_i)} \right).$$

The use of the log-trapeze method is obviously good if you benchmark it against a decreasing polyexponential. However, integrals are also to be computed when there is an absorption process, and on the rising part of such a curve this method may not provide a very good approximation. Mostly the log-trapeze method is therefore employed together with the trapeze method so that

- for an infusion, use the trapeze rule up to end of infusion and then the log-trapeze method

- for an extravascular administration, use the trapeze rule up to the point t_{max}, and then the log-trapeze rule.

A more refined method of this kind is Proost's method [4], which has an internal algorithm to decide for each interval if the trapeze or logtrapeze method should be used. It looks at the curvature by computing the expression

$$\frac{C_{i+1} - C_i}{t_{i+1} - t_i} - \frac{C_{i-1} - C_i}{t_{i-1} - t_i}.$$

If this is positive at a point, we use the log-linear approximation in the interval $[t_{i-1}, t_i]$, otherwise the linear.

To see what the difference is between using the trapeze method and the log-trapeze method, we compare the ratio of the latter to the former:

$$\frac{\frac{C_{i+1} - C_i}{\ln(C_{i+1}/C_i)} (t_{i+1} - t_i)}{\frac{C_{i+1} + C_i}{2} (t_{i+1} - t_i)} = \frac{2(\theta - 1)}{(\theta + 1) \ln \theta}, \quad \text{where} \quad \theta = C_{i+1}/C_i.$$

We see that the ratio only depends on how large the fall in plasma concentration is over the interval. We find, for instance, that if there is a 90% fall, the area ratio is 0.7, but if the fall is 40% the area ratio is only a little less than one.

The lesson from this is that since large areas are those for which a large relative difference matters most, sampling times should be chosen in a way that there are no numerically large falls over a sample interval, and these should be smaller the larger the concentration is. When only small concentrations remain, during the terminal elimination phase longer intervals can be used since the contribution to the total integral should be small and therefore the difference between these two methods should not have any practical consequences.

Errors in the estimate of the terminal elimination rate will influence the estimate of the PK parameters. So when we want to compute PK parameters for different administrations, we should not let differences in this estimated rate lead to differences in integral based parameters – at least not unless there is some good reason for it (as when one administration shows a flip-flop phenomenon). If we have an intravenous administration, we therefore may estimate the terminal elimination rate from this administration and then use that whenever we compute the extrapolated parts of various integrals. If we have two oral administrations, it is strongly recommended that a common terminal rate is used for both administrations, possibly by taking the (geometric) mean of two individually determined rates. There are exceptions to this rule: if one or both of the administrations has such a slow uptake that the absorption rate seriously influences the terminal elimination rate, one needs to balance the potential numerical problems in the estimation against this. When considerably different doses are given (or absorbed) we must consider the risk that the terminal phase is added too soon to the lower dose curve, i.e., attached to too large concentrations, resulting in a serious overestimation of the total area for that dose.

3.4 Numerical deconvolution

Deconvolution is the problem of solving a convolution equation. For example, if we know the plasma profile $G(t)$ after having given a unit bolus dose, and measure the plasma profile $C(t)$ after an extravascular administration, we know that

$$C(t) = (a * G)(t),$$

where $a(t)$ is the absorption rate from the extravascular site. In order to assess the absorption rate we need to solve this equation for $a(t)$. A numerical method for doing so is described in this section.

Assume, as in the previous section, that we have data $(t_i, C_i), i = 0, \ldots, n$ and $(s_i, G_i), i = 0, \ldots, m$, where measurement times may differ, but $t_0 = s_0 = 0$. We now approximate $a(t)$ with a step-function such that

$$a(t) = a_i, \quad t_{i-1} \le t \le t_i.$$

Under this assumption we have that $C(t_j)$ equals

$$\int_0^{t_j} G(t_j - s)a(s)\, ds = \sum_{i=1}^{j} \int_{t_{i-1}}^{t_i} G(t_j - s)a_i\, ds = \sum_{i=1}^{j} a_i \int_{t_j - t_i}^{t_j - t_{i-1}} G(s)\, ds.$$

If we therefore introduce the notation

$$I_{i,j}^{k,l} = \int_{t_i - t_j}^{t_k - t_l} G(s)\, ds,$$

we arrive at a linear system

$$
\begin{pmatrix} C_1 \\ C_2 \\ \cdots \\ C_n \end{pmatrix} = \begin{pmatrix} I_{1,1}^{1,0} & 0 & 0 & 0 & \cdots & 0 \\ I_{2,1}^{2,0} & I_{2,1}^{2,2} & 0 & 0 & \cdots & 0 \\ I_{3,1}^{3,0} & I_{3,2}^{3,1} & I_{3,2}^{3,3} & 0 & \cdots & 0 \\ & & & & \ddots & \\ \cdots & \cdots & \cdots & \cdots & & \cdots \\ I_{n,1}^{n,0} & I_{n,2}^{n,1} & I_{n,2}^{n,3} & I_{n,3}^{n,4} & \cdots & I_{n,n-1}^{n,n} \end{pmatrix} \begin{pmatrix} a_1 \\ a_2 \\ \cdots \\ a_n \end{pmatrix}.
$$

After choosing a method (as discussed in the previous section) to compute the integrals $I_{i,j}^{k,l}$ from the available data (s_i, G_i), we can solve this system to obtain a step-function approximation of the absorption profile $a(t)$.

3.5   Population average vs. subject-specific approach

When describing plasma profiles, mean values can be used. However, values below LOQ cannot simply be considered missing when computing these mean values, since they carry information. It is therefore important that trailing missing values, due to values below LOQ, are replaced with estimates, based on mono-exponentials using the estimated terminal elimination rate discussed in the previous section. Also other values below LOQ need to be filled in with an appropriate algorithm.

When computing mean values, it is preferable to compute geometric means. Much of the variability resides in dosing, at least from an extravascular site, which is a multiplicative factor to the plasma concentration, and by taking the geometric mean, we get the product of the geometric mean of doses and the geometric mean of dose one response curves (assuming linear kinetics).

It is important to know what a mean value curve represents. Its value at time t represents what the plasma concentration is expected to be, if we take one sample at that time for a randomly chosen individual after having dosed according to the schedule used. There is a potentially important difference between this mean curve and an individual curve. In order to illustrate the difference, assume a situation with a first order absorption profile and a one-compartment model such that all individuals in the world have the same plasma concentration curve, except that there is a time-lag until absorption starts. But assume that this time-lag varies substantially between individuals, so that the absorption starts much later for some individuals as compared to for others.

This is illustrated in Figure 3.2, in which we have shown five typical subject profiles, the middle of which is thicker than the others. This is a *mean parameter curve*, in this case the subject profile you get if you take as lag-time the mean value of all individual lag-times. It looks like the other curves and lies in

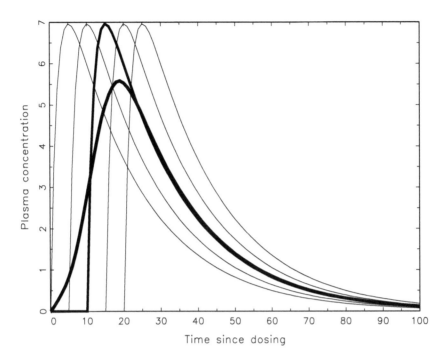

FIGURE 3.2: The difference between a mean curve and a mean parameter
curve

the middle of the family. The other thick curve is the *mean curve*, the curve
obtained by taking the means of all the other (not only the five shown, but
from the whole population). It looks quite different, and does not resemble an
individual curve. But it tells us what the mean plasma concentration should
be, if we fix a time point and sample many individuals at that time point.
This curve is the population average curve, and describing it is the *population
average approach* to data analysis. The mean parameter curve represents the
subject specific approach to data analysis.

Strictly speaking the difference between the mean parameter curve and
the mean curve makes most sense if we discuss a NONMEM application, in
which there is a clear meaning of the former. But we can think of a mean
parameter curve as "the most typical individual curve", obtained from "an
average individual".

3.6 A real example

3.6.1 Description of data

Treatment with an inhaled glucocorticosteroid (GCS) is important for most asthmatics. There are quite a few of these inhaled GCSs on the market, in different inhalation devices, and we studied the PK properties of two of them, budesonide and fluticasone proprionate. These two GCS have different physio-chemical properties in terms of solubility and how lipophilic they are, with fluticasone being ten times more lipophilic than budesonide. It is therefore of interest to compare their pharmacokinetic profiles. Data consists of plasma concentrations both after a 10 minute intravenous infusion and after a single inhalation using different inhalation devices, Turbuhaler®for budesonide and Discus®for fluticasone. The single dose administration was followed by a seven day multiple dosing period on each of these treatments, with twice daily administrations with the respective inhaler.

The data we discuss are taken from two different clinical studies, first discussed in [3]. Our data do not include all data of the two studies (two inhalers for fluticasone were studied in one of the studies). One of the studies was in healthy volunteers, the other in mild asthmatics. Also, the numerical methods used here differ in some details, like integration method, from what was used in [3], so the numbers reported here are at some places slightly different from those previously reported.

3.6.2 Determination of terminal elimination half-life

In order to compute standard PK parameters after a single dose, either an intravenous or an extravascular administration, we need an estimate of the plasma concentration curve all the way to infinity. This means that we need an extrapolation from the last measured time point onwards. This is done by determining a terminal elimination rate and then doing the extrapolation with a mono-exponential based on that, anchored at the last point measured. Since we have, for each drug, an intravenous administration, we use the terminal elimination rate estimated from those data when we compute all integrals, also those for other administrations.

Figure 3.3 shows in the top row the plasma concentrations after the infusion administration of the two drugs on a log-scale. In order to obtain linear approximation of the terminal part, we use the algorithm discussed in Section 3.2, but using only data obtained 6 hours or later after dosing. This is because there is sufficiently rich data for the estimate there, and there is always a risk with any numeric algorithm that it will interpret data in an inappropriate way. If, e.g., we have a slight bend at the end, the algorithm may find a long line that is steeper than the last part, and such a risk we want

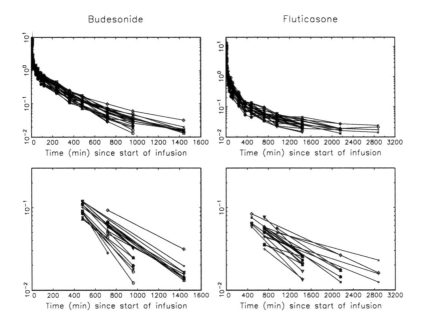

FIGURE 3.3: Intravenous GCS data. The first row contains infusion data for the two drugs, the second row the log-linear approximations that determine individual λ_{el}:s

to minimize. The actual linear approximations are shown in the second row of Figure 3.3. However, each individual line must be compared to the data in order to decide how appropriate it is. We assume this is done and will use the terminal elimination rates indicated by the straight lines in the bottom row of Figure 3.3.

When comparing the terminal elimination rates for the two drugs visually, please note that the time scale differs for budesonide and fluticasone. Adjusting for that, we find that the terminal rates are larger for budesonide than for fluticasone. The actual half-lives obtained from them will be described and discussed in the next section.

3.6.3   Description of distribution and elimination

The geometric mean of the plasma concentrations, normalized to a common dose of 400 nmol, is shown in Figure 3.4. We see that these mean curves differ in their profiles with a much slower terminal elimination for fluticasone.

The potential risks with using mean curves as descriptors of pharmacokinetics behavior were discussed Section 3.5. However, in our case the shape of the mean curve and the mean parameter curve do not seem to differ much (imagine the mean curve in the swarm of individual curves in Figure 3.3), so

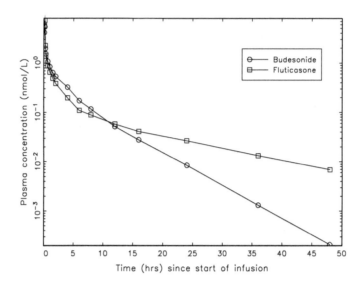

FIGURE 3.4: The geometric means of infusion data

a description of the mean curve may not be misleading.

However, for the rest of this discussion, we focus on individually computed basic PK parameters of distribution and elimination. Figure 3.5 shows the estimated parameters using the Proost method for integration. They are shown on a logarithmic scale, and since each point cluster appears reasonably symmetric about its median these plots justify that we summarize data in terms of geometric means and coefficient of variations.

Note that the variability of a particular PK parameter in Figure 3.5 has two components that add up. On one hand different individuals may have different true parameters (i.e., the parameter we would have computed if we had complete, continuous and error free measurements at our disposal to compute the parameter from). This is the inter-subject variability. But each of these true parameters are estimated from sparse data that are not error-free, using approximative integration methods. This means that if we estimate the same true parameter repeatedly we would get different numbers. An important contributor to this error is the estimate of the terminal elimination rate. This error component is the intra-subject variability. So the difference between an estimated parameter value and the population mean parameter value is the sum of the difference between the true individual parameter value and the population mean and the difference between the estimated parameter value for that individual and his/her true parameter value.

Figure 3.5 also shows the volume of the central space, V_c. This is estimated using equation 2.15, with a common rate estimate for the first phase for all individuals. We use a common rate estimate (geometric mean of individual

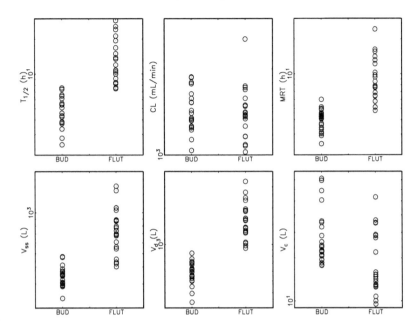

FIGURE 3.5: Individually computed PK parameters of distribution and elimination

ones) because this first phase is so short, that sample timing and precision
make individual estimates unprecise.

Table 3.1 gives a (geometric) mean summary of the parameters. In it we see
the similarities and differences of the two steroids clearly: they have the same
plasma clearance, around 1400 mL/min, whereas both MRT and V_{ss} are about
twice as large for fluticasone as for budesonide, and V_d and $t_{1/2}$ are almost
three times as large. The estimate of V_c is large enough (see next chapter)
to justify the assumption that we have central elimination for these drugs –
they are eliminated by metabolic breakdown in the liver and a central volume
of this size most probably includes both the liver and the kidneys. Also note
that the extrapolated area is almost three times larger for fluticasone than for
budesonide, due mainly to the longer $t_{1/2}$.

In summary, this means that fluticasone is distributed more extensively
than budesonide, whereas clearance is about the same. This is further illustrated in Figure 3.6, which shows estimates of how the volume curve $V(t)$ of
distribution evolves with time after an intravenous administration.

3.6.4   Absorption profiles

We will now study the absorption of the two steroids after a single dose from
the respective inhaler. The geometric mean values are shown in Figure 3.7.

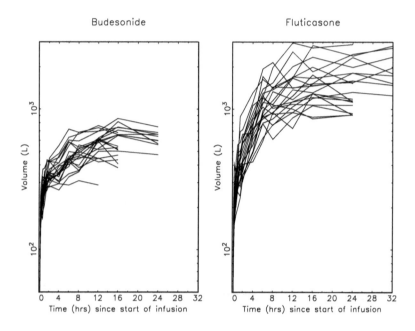

FIGURE 3.6: Individually computed volume curves

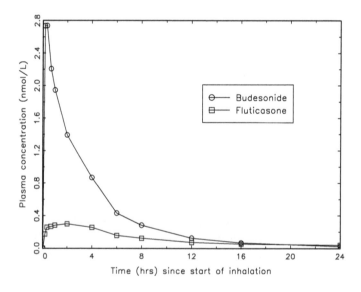

FIGURE 3.7: Geometric mean value curves for 24 hours after single dose administration

Table 3.1: Summary statistics of disposition and elimination parameters

Parameter	Budesonide		Fluticasone		Mean Ratio	
	mean	95% C.I.	mean	95% C.I.	ratio	95% C.I.
$t_{1/2}$ (h)	4.71	(4.11, 5.41)	12.9	(10.7, 15.6)	2.74	(2.19, 3.43)
CL (mL/min)	1431	(1327, 1543)	1405	(1281, 1541)	0.982	(0.875, 1.1)
MRT (h)	3.99	(3.62, 4.39)	8.77	(7.18, 10.7)	2.2	(1.77, 2.73)
V_{ss} (L)	342	(317, 369)	739	(620, 881)	2.16	(1.8, 2.6)
V_d (L)	584	(527, 646)	1570	(1342, 1836)	2.69	(2.24, 3.22)
V_c (L)	28.2	(23, 34.6)	18.4	(14.7, 23.1)	0.651	(0.485, 0.875)
AUC	280	(257, 304)	270	(246, 297)	0.966	(0.854, 1.09)
Extr. AUC (%)	3.04	(2.52, 3.66)	8.38	(6.98, 10.1)	2.76	(2.14, 3.55)

Since the drugs were inhaled, what is shown is their appearance in plasma. It means that the delay we see represents the transit time through lung tissue.

By inspection of the curves in Figure 3.7 we see that the absorption profile is somewhat different for the two drugs. For budesonide we see a sharp, high, early peak, whereas the absorption phase is much more prolonged for fluticasone. To describe this in numbers we compute a few key parameters that describe absorption. These are shown for each subject in Figure 3.8 and summarized statistically in Table 3.2.

Table 3.2: PK parameters describing absorption from the lungs after drug inhalation

Parameter	Budesonide		Fluticasone		Mean Ratio	
	mean	95% C.I.	mean	95% C.I.	ratio	95% C.I.
F (%)	40.6	(37.5, 43.9)	14.2	(12, 16.7)	0.35	(0.293, 0.418)
C_{max} (nmol/L)	3.57	(3.15, 4.03)	0.348	(0.304, 0.399)	0.0976	(0.0817, 0.117)
t_{max} (h)[a]	0.294	(0.214, 0.373)	1.79	(1.14, 2.44)	1.49	(0.857, 2.13)
MAT (h)[a]	0.902	(0.575, 1.23)	6.51	(5.52, 7.51)	5.61	(4.59, 6.63)

[a]: arithmetic mean and difference

We see that the fraction absorbed is about 3 times larger for budesonide than for fluticasone and the maximal concentration about 10 times larger, and that the mean absorption time is 5-6 hours longer for fluticasone than for budesonide.

Figure 3.9 shows the cumulative absorption curves, obtained by deconvolution. Among these there is, for each drug, a thicker curve which shows the absorption profile for the the first order absorption process based on the mean fraction absorbed and the MAT computed above. We see that this can play the role of a mean parameter curve for budesonide, indicating that the ab-

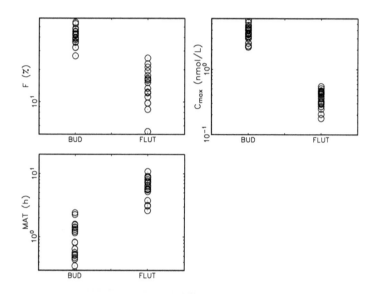

FIGURE 3.8: Individual PK parameters of absorption

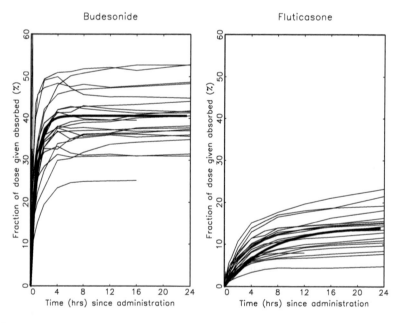

FIGURE 3.9: Deconvoluted absorption profiles. Thick lines are first order processes based on F and MAT.

sorption process is at least close to being first order. However, for fluticasone the deconvoluted absorption curves do not fit the thick curve well. Instead there appear to be two phases: a relatively fast first phase, followed by a much slower second phase. We do not investigate or discuss this observation further.

3.6.5   Accumulation at multiple dosing

Next we want to compare the data in steady state with the single-dose data, and how well the predictions we can make from single-dose data about steady state data turn out. As already pointed out, the assumption here is that the dose absorbed is the same after each administration. In this study the dosing interval was every 12th hour; so in Figure 3.10 we show the geometric means of 0–12 hour plasma concentrations after a single dose inhalation (the same data we discussed in the previous section) and after seven days of dosing.

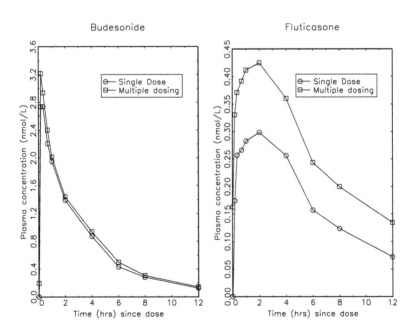

FIGURE 3.10: Single dose and multiple dose geometric mean 0-12 hour data for the two treatments

There are a few things to note. First, the start and end-values for the multiple dosing curves are almost on the same level, justifying the hypothesis that we are at least close to steady state. Second, we see that for budesonide the two curves almost coincide, with the multiple dosing curve possibly slightly above the single dose curve, whereas for fluticasone there is a larger discrepancy – or, in PK terms, drug accumulation. By computing the ratio of the geometric means, we get estimates of the geometric mean of the accumulation ratio, R_{ac} as a function of time, as shown in Figure 3.11

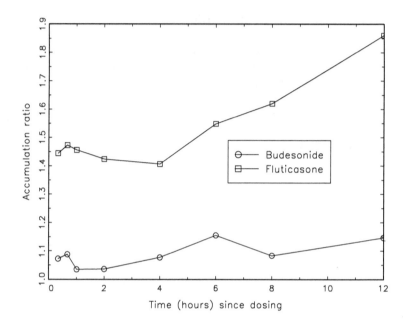

FIGURE 3.11: Accumulation ratio as a function of time for the two treatments

We supplement this with the AUC based accumulation ratio in Table 3.3 which contains the geometric means and mean ratios with confidence intervals, both for the predicted version based on single dose curves and for the observed version. Note that the variability is much smaller for the predicted version, since the numerator and the denominator in that case are determined from the same plasma concentration curve. The actual accumulation ratio, however, has numerator and denominator estimated from two different plasma concentration curves and can therefore be expected to have a larger variability.

When estimating the terminal elimination half-life, we pointed out the risk that we in fact miss a late, slower phase, because of insufficient measurement time or a too high LOQ. One crude way to find out if we have missed something important in that respect is to look at the accumulation data at the end of a dosing interval (12 hours). If we assume that the only contribution to this is

Table 3.3: Predicted and actual accumulation ratio

Parameter	Budesonide mean	Budesonide 95% C.I.	Fluticasone mean	Fluticasone 95% C.I.	Mean Ratio ratio	Mean Ratio 95% C.I.
Predicted accumulation	1.11	(1.08, 1.13)	1.65	(1.56, 1.74)	1.49	(1.41, 1.57)
Actual accumulation	1.08	(0.956, 1.22)	1.51	(1.34, 1.71)	1.40	(1.18, 1.65)

from a terminal phase, we can use the observation in equation 3.1 to compute a terminal elimination rate from the observed accumulation ratio at 12 hours post-dose. For our data this computation identifies approximative terminal half-lives of 11.9 and 6.1 hours for fluticasone and budesonide, respectively. These are fairly close to what our mean estimates were above.

3.7 Chapter epilogue: Pharmacokinetics in drug development

We end this chapter with a short discussion on which the key pharmacokinetics questions are in drug development and how and when they usually are addressed. The precise timing for these investigations in a drug development project depends on the availability of a reliable assay method that allows plasma concentrations to be measured. The assumption here is that the assay already is in place before the drug is given to a human for the first time. What we describe is a typical small-molecule project with a new chemical entity about which very little is known of how it is handled by the human body. The PK program aims at gathering information on absorption, distribution, metabolism, and excretion (abbreviated ADME) of the drug.

In order to start studies in humans, one needs an approved Investigational New Drug (IND) application. The foundation of this IND is an animal toxicology programme which is designed to identify toxicities that may appear in humans. Within this programme, PK information in the animals may help in defining an acceptable exposure limit in humans and therefore an appropriate starting dose when the drug is given to man for the first time.

The first clinical study that is made is typically a Single Ascending Dose (SAD) study. In such a study single doses are given to subjects (often healthy volunteers) which are then followed by measuring, among other things, adverse events, routine laboratory determinations, vitals signs, and heart effects. This is done in order to assess whether a particular dose is tolerable or not and, if it is, allows us to increase the dose. Such a study is the important first step in drug development and allows us to later study repeated dosing.

When doing the SAD study we may take the opportunity to study plasma concentrations of single doses. At this stage, the administration form is usually not an intravenous infusion but an oral formulation of some sort (a solution, a suspension, or even a tablet). It allows us to compute various PK parameters, but we do not know how much of the drug was actually taken up by the body. Therefore parameters like clearance and volumes can only by estimated up to a bioavailability factor. But what we can do, and this may be our only chance in a drug development programme to do that, is to study how AUC (i.e., $I(C)$) depends on the dose. As discussed in Chapter 2 this should be proportional to the given dose if the kinetics is linear. So we study the dose-AUC relationship in order to find out if there are signs of non-linearity, like capacity limited elimination. Note, however, that if we study non-intravenous administrations, there is the possibility that the bioavailability varies between doses, so that a non-linear appearance of the curve does not really reflect the systemic pharmacokinetics events. In fact, the shape of the non-linearity gives some indication on where it may arise. If AUC increases faster than proportionally to dose it is probably elimination that is non-linear; if AUC increases slower than proportionally to dose the most likely explanation is a decreasing bioavailability with increasing dose.

We can also use the PK to predict what plasma concentrations we should obtain when we give multiple doses. Such a study, a Multiple Ascending Dose (MAD) study, is typically the next study that is made. Like the SAD study it is primarily a tolerability study, but we may take the opportunity to study the pharmacokinetics after multiple dosing. The idea is to study the tolerability of the drug in steady state, so the study allows us to compare, for instance, the AUC over a dosing interval in steady state with that of a single dose administration. As discussed in Section 2.4, these two should be equal if we have linear kinetics, so this comparison is a test for that.

In addition to this, more focussed PK studies are usually needed. In such studies, we typically may give an intravenous infusion which allows us to address the systemic kinetics without complications due to absorption and we may take the opportunity to estimate the absorption process of a particular formulation by giving the same subject an intravenous administration and an oral administration on different occasions. A key information from such a study is the absolute bioavailability of the oral formulation.

Another question that comes early in a typical drug development programme is the question of whether there is a difference in the bioavailability of the drug when given with or without food. This can be done by comparing the AUC from subjects given a high fat breakfast on one occasion and a low fat breakfast at a different occasion in a special study. It can also be appended to the MAD study.

In addition to this, special studies may be needed in particular patient groups, like those with renal insufficiency or liver disease. Also very small studies need to be conducted that sample blood after drug administration. This is used to identify possible metabolites of the drug. When a new drug is given to patients, there is always a risk that a patient takes another drug at the same time which may share some metabolic pathway with the new drug. This could lead to changes in the PK behavior for either or both of the drugs, which is why such drugs need to be identified. If there is such an interaction, it may call for a warning on how to use the new drug. To assess the need for this, special drug-drug interaction studies where the drugs are given together may need to be performed.

Much of this information is typically obtained in rather small groups of subjects, often in healthy volunteers. To get information on the variability of PK parameters in patient groups one often uses an approach that among pharmacokineticists is called *population kinetics*. This means that in clinical studies in patients, where the effect of the drug is studied, one also takes a few samples of plasma concentrations of the drug. Then a model, built from the rich data studies discussed above, is applied to those data, using a NonLinear Mixed Effects Model (NONMEM) approach of analysis to the data. Appropriately parameterized this model gives information on the population variability in some key PK parameters. However, this type of analysis is outside the scope of this book – it is essentially built up by combining compartment models discussed later with the general estimation process NONMEM. It is enough to say that there is some confusion about the term population kinetics: its natural interpretation seems to be the study of pharmacokinetics in some (patient) population. It seems, however, often to be used as a descriptor for the NONMEM estimation method when applied to pharmacokinetic data.

During drug development, the drug formulation often changes with time. One may start out with a solution or suspension for the first studies but then develop some kind of tablet for oral use. When carrying information obtained with one formulation to another formulation, one has to do a *bioequivalence study*. If we want to replace formulation A with formulation B, this means that we take a single dose of each (at different occasions) and study the plasma profiles. What we need to assure ourselves is that the rates and extents of absorption are similar. This is, by a regulatory contract, studied by comparing AUC and C_{max} (and t_{max}) for the two formulations. The criterion that is universally accepted in this situation is that if the mean AUC ratio has a 90% confidence interval contained within the interval (0.80, 1.25), then we can consider the two formulations to be exchangeable (so that the data obtained on A can be used for B). If the doses are not the same, we have to compare dose corrected PK parameters (AUC/D and C_{max}/D). Note that this statistical analysis is made on the logarithm of the AUC and C_{max}.

Chapter 4

Physiological aspects on pharmacokinetics

4.1 Some physiological preliminaries

In this chapter we will discuss pharmacokinetics from a physiological perspective in order to better understand the nature of the pharmacokinetic models we have discussed so far and will discuss further in Chapter 5. This includes that we mathematically build a pharmacokinetics model that reflects at least parts of the physiology, and then analyze this model with the standard PK methods discussed so far.

About 2/3 of the human body consists of water. Adipose tissue contains only about 10% water, so the more fat you carry, the smaller this fraction will be. About 2/3 of the water is located within cells, the rest makes up the *ExtraCellular Fluid* (ECF) from which the nutrients needed by the cell are taken up and into which waste products are deposited. This includes oxygen and carbon-dioxide for cell respiration. The ECF is divided into plasma - the fluid of the vascular system - which is about 20% of it, and the interstitial fluid located in tissue spaces. Note that blood contains both ECF (plasma) and intracellular fluid, most of the latter within the red blood cells (also called erythrocytes). The volume ratio of red blood cells to total blood is called the *hematocrit*.

In order to measure the volumes of the different spaces, we need to find appropriate substances to give and then measure concentrations of them. In order to determine the plasma volume we need a molecule that stays in the plasma (a dye called Evans blue can be used), in order to measure the total extracellular space we need a substance that enters it but does not enter cells (labelled inulin, a sugar produced by plants in order to store energy, can be used). To find the intracellular space we need to find the total volume of body water, which can be done with heavy water, and then subtract the ECF volume.

Intracellular water is contained within the cell by the cell membrane, which is built up of a double phospholipid layer with large molecules like proteins embedded in it. Some of these are receptors that may be the target of our drug, something to be discussed in Chapter 6. The cell membrane is semi-permeable in that it allows easy passage of some molecules but not of others, depending on molecular size and its physio-chemical properties. Lipophilic substances, like oxygen and CO_2, pass easily through the walls, whereas hydrophilic substances, including water, need to find pores in the cell membrane to pass through, and therefore can only enter if they are small enough. This means that there is an osmotic pressure over the cell membrane. The term *osmosis*[1] refers to the motion over a semi-permeable membrane which makes, for instance, water move towards the side with the overall higher particle concentration. In general the different fluids in the body are separated by semi-permeable membranes. As a result the molecule composition of different aqueous spaces differ.

An assembly of similarly specialized cells and their derivatives (intercellular substances) is called a *tissue*. Tissue classification, which refers to cell type, not function, includes epithelial tissues, which cover all external and internal surfaces of the body, muscle tissue, comprising of all contractile elements, nerve tissue, and connective and supporting tissues (bones, cartilage). The latter are found in the locomotor apparatus, in blood vessels, and in supporting structures. Cells of these basic tissues are in different ways combined to form larger, *functional* units which we call organs. We will not distinguish clearly between organ and tissue, instead we will use the two words interchangeably.

The vascular system is a network of tubes through which the blood flows, driven by the heart. Vessels in which the blood is leaving the heart are called arteries, and vessels that carry blood to the heart are called veins. These are connected within tissues by smaller vessels, capillaries. It is in the capillaries that the exchange of molecules between plasma and tissues occur. These capillaries also have different permeability properties in different tissues, with one extreme being the blood-brain barrier that hardly lets many substances through.

In the vascular system there are two serially connected but synchronized pumps, the right heart and the left heart, which separate the major, systemic circulation from the minor, pulmonary circulation. Arteries in the systemic circulation carry oxygen-rich blood and veins carry CO_2-rich blood, whereas the opposite is true in the pulmonary circulation. The pulmonary circulation contains only one organ, the lungs, whereas the systemic circulation features the rest of the body organs, most of them connected in parallel. Some organs are serially connected but taken together constitute a larger organ that is connected in parallel with the others. The most important example is the intestines and the liver, as will be discussed in more detail in Section 4.4. The flow (mL/min) of the blood in a particular vessel is given by the ratio

---

[1]The passage of pure solvent from a solution of lesser to one of greater solute concentration when the two solutions are separated by a membrane which selectively prevents the passage of solute molecules, but is permeable to the solvent

between the blood pressure, produced by the heart, and the vascular resistance determined by its diameter. The blood flow differs between organs.

The blood pressure leads to a hydrostatic pressure ΔP over the capillary walls. Opposing this is the osmotic pressure $\Delta\Pi$, so we get a net filtration rate which is proportional to the pressure difference $\Delta P - \Delta\Pi$, with a proportionality coefficient that differ between tissues. Since the arterial pressure is larger than the venous one, the net flow is into the interstitial space in the beginning and back into the blood at the end of the capillaries. There is normally a slight excess in fluid efflux compared to influx. This extra fluid is removed from the interstitial space by the lymph system and returned to the blood.

In the coming sections of this chapter, we will first discuss drug kinetics from a water compartment perspective in order to discuss the interpretation of the distribution volume of a drug. After that we will consider drug transport through the circulatory system and how it enters and leaves the body organs. This will include a discussion of the clearance concept but also help us understand the connection between the standard NCA model and our perception of what happens to the drug in the body.

4.2 Distribution volume

4.2.1 Protein binding

When small molecules like inorganic ions and hormones enter the blood stream they usually become more or less bound to proteins in it. Such proteins are called transport or carrier proteins. The most well-known example is perhaps hemoglobin (which transports O_2 and CO_2), a protein found within the red blood cells. The second most important example is albumin which can bind a large variety of substances. The extent of protein binding varies from almost nothing (e.g., urea) up to almost 100% (e.g., thyroxine). Alcohol is not bound to plasma proteins at all. Protein binding is not confined to plasma but occurs in other aqueous compartments as well. However, proteins seldom pass over the membranes separating these compartments, so in order for a molecule to pass from one water compartment to another, it has to be unbound.

Most synthetic drugs also bind to proteins. Many are designed to bind to a specific protein either on a cell surface or within a cell, a protein then called a receptor. Typically they also bind to transport proteins in the blood. Note that it is only unbound molecules that bind to receptors and therefore can have a pharmacological effect.

In order to describe the process of protein binding, consider a particular protein P. Let P_0 denote the total protein concentration. Denote the drug with D and its free concentration by $[D]$ (later this will be denoted C_u). Then we have that

$$[P] + [DP] = P_0,$$

where $[P]$ is the concentration of unbound protein and $[DP]$ the concentration of the drug-protein complex. The chemical reaction

$$D + P \underset{k_{-1}}{\overset{k_1}{\rightleftharpoons}} DP$$

and the law of mass action then implies the differential equation

$$[DP]' = k_1[D][P] - k_{-1}[DP].$$

This reaction is usually very fast (milliseconds) and we can therefore assume that it is always in equilibrium, i.e., $[DP]' = 0$, so that

$$[DP] = K_a[D][P], \quad K_a = \frac{k_1}{k_{-1}}. \tag{4.1}$$

The constant K_a is called the *association constant* of the binding, and measures the *affinity* of the binding. A direct consequence of formula 4.1 is that the fraction of unbound drug is given by

$$f_u = \frac{[D]}{[D] + [DP]} = \frac{1}{1 + K_a[P]}. \tag{4.2}$$

For many proteins that occur in great abundance, for instance, albumin, we have that $[P] \approx P_0$, also in the presence of drug.

A clinically important consequence of formula 4.2 is that if the total concentration of transport protein to bind to decreases, the fraction of unbound drug will increase. Since this fraction is the biologically active part, this may have consequences for what dose of the drug we should give. There are different reasons why P_0 could decrease. Other substances, e.g., other drugs, may compete for the same binding sites. It can be low also as a consequence of some disease, for instance, in the liver. Plasma proteins are typically synthesized in the liver.

Example 4.1
Phenytoin is an old anti-epileptic drug for which the therapeutic window is 10–20 mg/L. It is substantially bound to plasma albumin and at a normal albumin level of 44 g/L we have a free fraction of 0.1. Now consider a patient with an albumin level of 20 g/L for whom the average concentration of phenytoin is 6 mg/L. Is this a sub-therapeutic concentration?

To answer that question, note that it is the unbound drug that has effect, and its therapeutic window is 1–2 mg/L. From the data above we can determine K_a from equation 4.2, obtained at normal albumin levels, giving us $K_a = 9/44$. Therefore the free fraction at an albumin level of 20 g/L is $f_u = 1/(1 + 20 \cdot 9/44) = 0.2$, so 20% of the observed total concentration of 6 mg/L is unbound, leading to a free concentration of 1.2 mg/L. This is within the therapeutic window for free drug. ⬚

4.2.2 Volume decomposition

The total body water volume is about 42 liters. How, then, can the volume we measure as, say, V_{ss}, at times be hundreds of liters? How can it ever by more than 42 liters? In this section we set out to explain this in some detail. The discussion assumes a *Gedankenexperiment*, in which we have administered drug to a body for which we have turned off the elimination mechanism and then waited until the drug is in equilibrium throughout the body. There is no net transport anywhere.

In order to explain the idea we first assume that we can divide the total body water into two spaces, each of which the drug is well mixed in. The first we call the central space, with volume V_c and concentration C_c. The second we call the peripheral space with volume V_p and concentration C_p. The total body volume is then $V = V_c + V_p$. But that is not the volume we measure. What we measure is the total amount of drug $(V_cC_c + V_pC_p)$ divided with the only concentration we can see, C_c. This means that

$$V_{ss} = V_c + \frac{C_p}{C_c}V_p.$$

The ratio of concentrations here is called the *partition coefficient*[2]

$$K_p = \frac{C_p}{C_c}$$

for the peripheral space (relative the central one), and using it we rewrite the formula for V_{ss} as

$$V_{ss} = V_c + K_pV_p.$$

We can interpret K_p as follows. Assume that bound drug cannot leave its space, while unbound drug can pass freely between spaces, so that the concentration of unbound drug, C_u, is the same in the two spaces; see Figure 4.1. Let $f_{u,c}, f_{u,p}$ denote the fraction of unbound drug in the central space and peripheral space respectively. We then have that

$$C_u = f_{u,c}C_c = f_{u,p}C_p.$$

---

[2]In this section there is a varying use of the index p. In K_p it refers to partition, whereas as index to C or V it has so far referred to peripheral (space). Later on it will refer to plasma. Hopefully the context clarifies what is at hand.

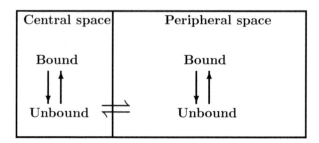

FIGURE 4.1: The distribution of drug is at equilibrium determined by protein binding, assuming only unbound drug passes through barriers

It follows that $K_p = f_{u,c}/f_{u,p}$, which gives us the equation

$$V_{ss} = V_c + \frac{f_{u,c}}{f_{u,p}}V_p.$$

This shows that it is the fraction of unbound drug that defines the volume we measure. A drug which is more strongly bound outside the central space than in the central space will have a larger apparent volume than one that is more weakly bound. Note that the amount of drug outside the central compartment over the amount in it is given by

$$\frac{V_pC_p}{V_cC_c} = \frac{V_p}{V_c}\frac{f_{u,c}}{f_{u,p}}.$$

The lesson from this is the relation between fraction unbound and apparent volume. The assumption of a homogenous peripheral space may not be fully correct from a physiological perspective, so we will soon proceed with the ideas above in a more realistic setting. First an example related to the discussion above.

Example 4.2
The blood volume V_b is the sum of its plasma volume V_p and the volume of red blood cells, V_{RBC},

$$V_b = V_p + V_{RBC}.$$

The amount of a particular drug in blood is then equal to the amount in plasma and the amount in the erythrocytes:

$$V_bC_b = V_pC_p + V_{RBC}C_{RBC} = C_p(V_p + K_pV_{RBC}),$$

where K_p is the partition coefficient for red blood cells relative plasma. If we only measure plasma concentration, the distribution volume would be $V_{ss} =$

$V_p + K_p V_{RBC}$. Since the hematocrit is defined by $H = V_{RBC}/V_b$, we also find that the ratio of blood concentration to plasma concentration is determined by the hematocrit and the partition coefficient as

$$\frac{C_b}{C_p} = 1 - H + K_p H. \tag{4.3}$$

This observation is important if we, for instance, want to relate blood clearance to plasma clearance. In fact, we have that

$$CL_b = \frac{C_p}{C_b} CL_p.$$

▯

Referring to the introductory overview of physiology, we divide the body water into *intracellular* and *extracellular* water. These aqueous compartments are separated by semi-permeable membranes. A special organ is the blood vessels, for which there is a wall of endothelial cells enclosing the blood. Blood consists of plasma (extracellular fluid) and intracellular water (within blood cells). The rest of the extracellular fluid consists of interstitial fluid that is within organs, outside cells. As a first approximation we therefore have two types of membranes to consider: those that make up the walls of blood vessels separating plasma from interstitial fluid, and the cell membranes separating interstitial fluid from intracellular fluid. A special case of the latter is the plasma-blood cell membrane. The following table gives an indication of the volumes involved for humans:

Extracellular water	13-16 L
Plasma	3 L
Interstitial fluid	10–13 L
Intracellular water	25–28 L
Trans-cellular water[1]	0.7–2L

[1] excretion of different kinds - intestinal, nose etc

Focussing on these three compartments: plasma, denoted by index p, the interstitial fluid, denoted by index ec (referring to extracellular minus plasma), and the intracellular space, denoted by index ic, we can, in complete analogy with what we did above, divide the available mass up on the three compartments. Assuming that the concentration of unbound drug is the same everywhere, we get

$$V_{ss} = V_p + \frac{f_{u,p}}{f_{u,ec}} V_{ec} + K_{p,ic} V_{ic}. \tag{4.4}$$

This is a simple formula, completely analogous to the one obtained when we only divided the available water into a central and a peripheral compartment.

It is not necessarily a good approximation of the actual volume. In fact, there is a refined version for very abundant transport proteins, like albumin, which is discussed in Box 4.1.

Example 4.3

The drug warfarin is bound in plasma to 99% and has a volume of distribution of 7.7 liters. Assume that the amount of plasma proteins that warfarin bind to suddenly decreases so much that the bound warfarin fraction decreases to 90%, what would then the volume of distribution be?

Dividing body water up into plasma and tissue, with indices p and t, we have the formula

$$V_{ss} = V_p + \frac{f_{u,p}}{f_{u,t}} V_t,$$

and inserting $V_p = 3, V = 7.7$ and $f_{u,p} = 0.01$ into that we find that $V_t/f_{u,t} = 470$ liters. If we assume that the fraction of free drug in the tissues is unchanged when we lose plasma proteins we find that with $f_{u,p} = 0.10$ instead we would have a volume of distribution of

$$V_{ss} = 3 + 0.1 \cdot 470 = 50 \text{ liters.}$$

However, warfarin binds to albumin, and if the reason for the protein loss is a liver disease, we would find a proportional drop in albumin in all compartments. Then using the albumin formula in Box 4.1 instead, we first get the relation

$$7.7 = 7.2 + 0.01(7.8 + 27/f_{u,ic})$$

from which we find that $f_{u,ic} = 0.64$. Holding this number fixed, the volume of distribution in the liver disease situation would be

$$V_{ss} = 7.2 + 0.10(7.8 + 27/0.64) = 12 \text{ liters.}$$

We see two very different predictions. But they are based on different hypotheses: in the first calculation the fraction unbound in the interstitial fluid was assumed unchanged, which is not the case in the second, so there is nothing contradictory in it. □

So far we have considered the intracellular space as one pool with a common concentration. That may not be true since different cell types may have different partition coefficients. This may force us to consider the total intracellular space as consisting of a collection of tissues whose cell membranes have different permeability to the drug. This means that we may need to divide the total intracellular volume V_{ic} into N sub-volumes $V_1, \ldots V_N$ with different partition coefficients, and a simple argument dividing amounts in the total intracellular space up between these tissues gives us

$$K_{p,ic} V_{ic} = K_{p,1} V_1 + \ldots + K_{p,N} V_N.$$

Box 4.1 An albumin formula

Albumin is an example of a protein to which drugs bind. It is found both in plasma and in the interstitial fluid in great abundance in both. For a drug that binds to such a protein, there is a refinement to equation 4.4, which we will now derive.

Assume, as before, that the free drug concentration C_u is the same everywhere. From equation 4.1 we have that $[DP]_p = C_u[P]_p$ and $[DP]_{ec} = C_u[P]_{ec}$ and from this we obtain that

$$\frac{[DP]_p}{[P]_p} = \frac{[DP]_{ec}}{[P]_{ec}}.$$

It follows that the concentration of drug-protein-complex in the interstitial fluid is proportional to the corresponding concentration in plasma:

$$[DP]_{ec} = [DP]_p \frac{[P]_{ec}}{[P]_p} \approx [DP]_p R \frac{V_p}{V_{ec}},$$

where we have introduced the constant

$$R = \frac{\text{amount extracellular protein}}{\text{amount plasma protein}}.$$

For albumin it is known that 55-60% of all albumin resides outside plasma from which we get an estimate $R \approx 1.4$. If we divide the amount of drug we have in the extracellular space ($V_{ec}C_{ec}$) into bound ($V_{ec}C_u$) and unbound drug ($V_{ec}[DP]_{ec}$), we get the relation

$$V_{ec}C_{ec} = V_{ec}C_u + V_{ec}[DP]_{ec} = V_{ec}f_{u,p}C_p + (1 - f_{u,p})C_p R V_p.$$

Insert this into equation 4.4 and rearrange slightly to get:

$$V_{ss} = V_p(1 + R) + f_{u,p}(V_{ec} - RV_p) + K_p V_{ic}.$$

For albumin this gives us the approximative formula

$$V_{ss} = 7.2 + 7.8 f_{u,p} + 27 \frac{f_{u,p}}{f_{u,ic}}.$$

Here we have used $R = 1.4$, a plasma volume of 3 liters, a total extracellular space of 15 liters (so that $V_{ec} = 12$) and an intracellular volume of 27 liters.

In summary, in steady state the drug is distributed over a volume $V = V_p + V_{ec} + V_1 + \ldots V_N$ but since we only get data from plasma, what we see is an apparent volume $V_{ss} = V_p + K_{p,ec}V_{ec} + K_{p,1}V_1 + \ldots K_{p,N}V_N$ for some N, where the partition coefficients are functions of protein binding in the tissues in question.

4.3 Events within an organ

4.3.1 Fick's principle

We will now add dynamics to the physiological picture, starting from the observation that the plasma we sample from is pumped around in the circulatory system. In fact, much of the discussion will be simpler if we consider not plasma concentration, but whole blood concentration. Some organs, like the liver and kidney, may try to eliminate the drug, while it may be temporarily stored in others. Fick's principle is the name in physiology of an observation that occurs in many sciences: at a particular point in the circulatory system, so much must leave that entered, minus what was eliminated or stored plus what was added. The statement is about flows. We will now look at different types of organs to see how Fick's principle can give us some insight into what happens to drugs in the body.

When we look at a part of the circulatory system, there are two conservation laws that must prevail:

conservation of volume the sum of blood flow entering must equal the sum of blood flows leaving the point

conservation of mass the amount of drug leaving must equal what entered minus what was lost, either eliminated or just stored in the organ, plus any new amount added from the outside.

We will denote amounts of drug by M and blood flow by Q. Concentrations will be blood concentrations, unless otherwise stated. If there is one vessel in and one vessel out, the flow in, Q_{in}, must equal the flow out, Q_{out}, provided there is no loss of water. Note that this does not quite apply to the kidneys, in which there is a small loss to the urine:

$$Q_{in} = Q_{out} + Q_U,$$

where Q_U is the urine flow. In fact, it does not quite apply to the liver either, because there is a loss to the bile. When discussing the liver we will ignore this loss to the bile, despite the independent interest it has in accounting for the enterohepatic cycle in which drug is excreted from the liver to the intestines, only to return.

As a preliminary application of the principles, Box 4.2 outlines two ways, used in the clinic, by which the cardiac output can be determined.

4.3.2 The organ transfer function

Consider an organ for which blood supply is through one ingoing and one outgoing vessel and in which there is no loss of water. Denote the blood flow in the ingoing and outgoing vessel with Q. Let C_{in} be the concentration of drug in the ingoing vessel and C_{out} the concentration in the outgoing one. Assuming a linear PK system we have a function $H(t)$ such that

$$C_{out} = H * C_{in}.$$

In fact, multiply this with Q and we have to the left the flow of drug out, whereas QC_{in} represents the flow of drug in. The function $H(t)$ is the fraction of drug which entered at time zero that leaves at time t. Thus the fraction of drug which enters the organ and actually leaves it is given by the integral $I(H)$. It follows that if the organ is non-eliminating, then $I(H) = 1$, and that $I(H) = 1 - E$ otherwise, where E is called the *extraction ratio* over the organ.

Note that if we put the system in steady state by applying a continuous infusion of drug on the ingoing vessel we have that $C_{out} = I(H)C_{in}$ and therefore that

$$E = \frac{C_{in} - C_{out}}{C_{in}},$$

so the extraction ratio is the ratio of rate of elimination to rate of presentation.

The function $H(t)/I(H)$ will be a probability density describing the transit time of the tissue. We therefore call $H(t)$ the transfer function of the tissue, and its Mean Transit Time is defined by

$$\text{MTT}(H) = \frac{E(H)}{I(H)}.$$

The function $H(t)$ can be obtained by measuring both C_{in} and C_{out}, and deconvolve the equation relating them. In the next section, we will see that if $H(t)$ is a simple mono-exponential function, the drug can be assumed to be well mixed in the tissue.

4.3.3 A well-stirred non-eliminating organ

Assume that our organ contains no internal barriers to the drug, so that it contains well-mixed drug with concentration C_T over a volume V_T. Assume first that the organ is non-eliminating and that the blood flow is Q. Then $M_T = V_T C_T$ is the amount of drug in the organ, and we have that

$$QC_{out} = QC_{in} - M'_T.$$

Box 4.2 Determination of cardiac output using Fick's principle

Here we will describe two methods to determine the cardiac output. The first is based on oxygen consumption in steady state, Q_{O_2}. This must equal the flow of new oxygen, which is given by the arterio-venous oxygen concentration difference $C_a - C_v$ times the cardiac output Q_c. So the formula we end up with is

$$Q_c(C_a - C_v) = Q_{O_2},$$

from which the cardiac output can be derived. Actual data can be obtained by noting that the pulmonary flow equals the cardiac output. C_v is measured in the pulmonary artery, whereas C_a can be measured in a peripheral artery. Oxygen consumption is measured by collecting and analyzing air breathed.

The second method of determining the cardiac output is by a dye-dilution technique. Choose a dye that is quickly and firmly bound to plasma proteins so that it leaves the blood stream only very slowly. Inject it as a bolus dose D in a vein which will carry it directly to the heart, and measure the concentration of the dye when it leaves the heart. We remove the molecules from the body as soon they appear. If $M(t)$ is the amount of drug in the body at time t, we then have $M'(t) = -Q_c C_a(t)$ and therefore

$$D = Q_c \int_0^\infty C_a(t)dt,$$

from which Q_c can be computed. The catch with this scheme is that we need to remove what is measured. In practice what is done instead is that the concentration curve $C_a(t)$ is measured, and when a small 'bump' starts to appear indicating recirculated dye, we fit a mono-exponential to the preceding data and extrapolate a dye concentration curve, representing only first pass of molecules at the site of measurement. And that is what is integrated under. Also, this means that we do not need to measure proximally in the aorta; any peripheral artery will do since the concentration is the same.

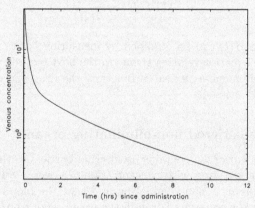

Organ	Volume (V_T) (mL)	Blood flow (Q) (mL/min)	Perfusion rate (Q/V_T) (mL/min/mL tissue)
Veins	3400	5330	1.57
Arteries	2100	5330	2.54
Liver	1400	1450	1.04
Kidneys	270	1170	4.33
GI tract	1200	880	0.73
Lungs	950	5330	5.61
Brain	1350	690	0.51
Muscles	30200	1050	0.03
Adipose tissue	18200	460	0.03
Skin	3400	510	0.15

Table 4.1: Blood flow and perfusion rate of main organs

We further assume that
$$C_{out} = C_T/K_p,$$
where K_p is the tissue partition coefficient. This assumption means that we assume that free drug instantly equilibrates between the tissue water and the water in the outgoing vessel. Inserting this into the equation and rearranging terms we get
$$V_T C_T' = Q(C_{in} - C_T/K_p). \tag{4.5}$$
If we start with no drug in the organ and keep C_{in} constant, we find that
$$C_T(t) = C_{in} K_p (1 - e^{-tQ/V_T K_p}).$$
Asymptotically the tissue concentration approaches $C_{in} K_p$, as it should, and the rate with which it does so is given by the *tissue rate constant*
$$k_T = \frac{Q}{V_T K_p}.$$
This number is built up from two numbers: K_p which is drug specific, and Q/V_T which is organ specific and called the perfusion rate of the organ. Table 4.1 contains a description of some set of plausible values for these physiological parameters for some key organs of the body. Note that arteries, veins and lungs have the cardiac output as blood flow and that numbers have been adjusted so that this equals the sum of the other organ flows.

We can note that equation 4.5 allows us to estimate K_p from non-steady state data: perfuse the organ with drug for a short time and measure drug concentration both in ingoing vessel and in the tissue. Integration of the equation then shows that
$$K_p = \frac{\int_0^\infty C_T(t)\, dt}{\int_0^\infty C_{in}(t)\, dt}.$$

The same equation 4.5 also tells us how we can estimate the tissue rate k_T for a particular organ. In fact if we integrate equation 4.5 after having substituted C_{out}/K_p for C_T we get

$$C_{out}(t) - C_{out}(0) = k_T \int_0^t (C_{in}(s) - C_{out}(s))ds.$$

If we choose a substance with a known K_p, and which is not eliminated in the organ in question, and put on a continuous administration (like an intravenous infusion) we asymptotically approach a steady state at which $C_{in}(\infty) = C_{out}(\infty)$. We can then estimate the organ perfusion rate from

$$\frac{Q}{V_T} = \frac{K_p C_{out}(\infty)}{\int_0^\infty (C_{in}(t) - C_{out}(t))\, dt}.$$

4.3.4   A well-stirred eliminating organ

With the same assumptions about the drug and organ as in the previous section, we now turn our attention to an organ that eliminates the drug. The two most important such organs are the liver and the kidneys. In the liver the drug is metabolized by enzymatic conversion to new molecules, possibly forming biologically active metabolites that could be of independent interest. The kidneys excrete some drugs.

It is only the free fraction of drug that is available for elimination, and we describe elimination using the concept of the *intrinsic clearance*, CL_{int}, of the tissue

$$\text{amount eliminated per time unit} = CL_{int}C_u.$$

Here C_u is the local free drug concentration. The intrinsic clearance is a clearance concept which addresses the ability of the tissue to eliminate the drug, free of constraints on blood flow and plasma binding issues. It is typically a function of C_u; if it is enzymatically converted by N different enzyme systems, we, for instance, have

$$CL_{int} = \sum_{i=1}^N \frac{v_{m,i}}{K_{m,i} + C_u},$$

see Box 4.3. At low free drug concentration CL_{int} is therefore approximately given by the sum $\sum_{i=1}^N v_{m,i}/K_{m,i}$ and the elimination rate is therefore (approximately) proportional to C_u.

Generalizing equation 4.5 to an eliminating organ we have the equation[3],

$$V_T C_T' = Q(C_{in} - C_{out}) - CL_{int}f_u C_{out}. \tag{4.6}$$

---

[3]In applying this equation to the liver we have to assume that drug from the two ingoing vessels, the hepatic artery and the portal vein, mix well before entering the liver, and also to ignore the bile flow

---

Box 4.3 Basic enzyme kinetics

Classical enzyme kinetics is described by the chemical reaction

$$S + E \underset{k_{-1}}{\overset{k_1}{\rightleftharpoons}} SE \overset{k_2}{\rightarrow} P + E,$$

where S denotes substrate, E enzyme and P denotes the conversion product. Note that the amount of enzyme is conserved. Written down as a system of differential equations we have

$$
\begin{aligned}
[S]' &= k_{-1}[SE] - k_1[S][E], & [S](0) &= S_0 \\
[E]' &= (k_{-1} + k_2)[SE] - k_1[S][E], & [E](0) &= E_0 \\
[SE]' &= k_1[S][E] - (k_{-1} + k_2)[SE], & [SE](0) &= 0 \\
[P]' &= k_2[SE], & [P](0) &= 0.
\end{aligned}
$$

If we note that $[E](t) + [SE](t) = E_0$, we find this system reduced to two non-linear differential equations

$$
\begin{aligned}
[S]' &= (k_1[S] + k_{-1})[SE] - k_1 E_0[S] \\
[SE]' &= k_1 E_0[S] - (k_1[S] + k_{-1} + k_2)[SE].
\end{aligned}
$$

At this stage there is often an assumption made, called a quasi-equilibrium hypothesis, namely that $[SE]' \approx 0$. Assuming this, we can solve $[SE]$ from the second equation and plug it into the first, to get the following equation for the velocity $-[S]'$ of the reaction:

$$-[S]' = \frac{k_2 E_0[S]}{k_1[S] + k_{-1} + k_2} = \frac{v_m}{K_m + [S]}[S],$$

where $K_m = (k_{-1} + k_2)/k_1$ and $v_m = E_0 k_2/k_1$.

We can note that

$$\frac{1}{-[S]'} = \frac{1}{v_m} + \frac{K_m}{v_m}\frac{1}{[S]}$$

which shows us a classical way to obtain the parameters K_m and v_m from data: plot the reciprocal of the velocity of the reaction versus the reciprocal of the substrate. Fit a straight line to the data and v_m is obtained as the reciprocal of the intercept and thereafter we obtain K_m from this and the slope of the line. This is the *Lineweaver-Burk* method of plotting the data.

Here the elimination term should actually be $CL_{int}C_{u,T}$, where $C_{u,T}$ is the free drug concentration in the tissue, but we have assumed this to be in equilibrium with the free concentration in the outgoing vessel, which is $f_u C_{out}$.

Assuming a constant CL_{int}, and if we apply a continuous infusion on the ingoing vessel, equation 4.6 implies that we in steady state will get the balance equation

$$QC_{out} = QC_{in} - CL_{int}f_u C_{out},$$

from which we get the extraction ratio of the organ as

$$E = \frac{f_u CL_{int}}{Q + f_u CL_{int}}. \tag{4.7}$$

It follows that the total blood clearance of the organ can be computed from

$$CL_{org} = Q \cdot E = \frac{Q f_u CL_{int}}{Q + f_u CL_{int}}.$$

The importance of this formula is that if we measure the extraction ratio E over the organ, we can use it to compute the intrinsic clearance. However, the expression relies heavily on the assumption that a drug mixed well in the tissue. For more comments on this, see Section 4.6

In clinical practice one distinguishes between low extraction substances (with E close to 0) and high extraction substances (with E close to 1). In the former case, $CL_{org} \approx f_u CL_{int}$ is virtually independent of the blood flow Q, whereas for the latter it is almost proportional to it ($CL_{org} \approx Q$). More importantly, for a drug with a low extraction ratio, the fraction free drug is important for the clearance.

Note that if we want to use CL_{org} in order to estimate the extraction ratio E, it is necessary to use the blood clearance, not the plasma clearance.

Still assuming a constant intrinsic clearance, we can rewrite equation 4.6 in terms of the extraction ratio instead as

$$V_T K_p C'_{out} = Q(C_{in} - C_{out}/(1 - E)). \tag{4.8}$$

This system is solved by the organ transfer function

$$C_{out} = H * C_{in}, \qquad H(t) = k_T e^{-k_T t/(1-E)}.$$

We see that $I(H) = 1 - E$ and that the mean transit time of the organ is

$$\mathrm{MTT}(H) = \frac{1 - E}{k_T} = \frac{V_T K_p (1 - E)}{Q}.$$

Another relevant concept in this situation is the *first pass effect* which applies, for instance, to a drug that is absorbed from the gastrointestinal tract and metabolized in the liver. Such a drug has to pass the liver before it can present itself at the sampling site in the circulatory system. The drug may also be metabolized by enzymes in the mucosa of the gastrointestinal tract, so some drug can be eliminated prior to reaching the liver. With obvious notation, the fraction of drug that is found in plasma is then

$$F = (1 - E_{GI})(1 - E_H).$$

The rest is destroyed before we ever can see it in plasma.

In order to keep the internal environment constant the body needs to excrete various metabolically produced waste products and substances ingested in excess of what the body needs. The chief organs for this are the kidneys. To understand what the components of the intrinsic clearance of the kidneys are, we need to know a little of the anatomy and physiology of the kidneys. Box 4.4 contain an ultra-brief outline of some key elements of relevance to us concerning its anatomy and physiology.

From Box 4.4 we see that the intrinsic clearance of the kidneys is made up of three components:

GFR is the glomerular filtration rate with which plasma water is filtered. It is about 125 mL/min.

Secretion is the capacity limited process which occurs if the substance is actively excreted.

Reabsorption is generally passive and occurs along the full nephron.

In all, this gives us an expression for the intrinsic clearance that can be written

$$CL_{int} = (1 - F_{reabs})(\text{GFR} + \frac{T_m}{K_m + C_u}),$$

where T_m represents a transport maximum and F_{reabs} of drug denotes the fraction that is reabsorbed from the tubules.

Note that only about one percent of what is filtered out with the glomerular filtration actually enters the urine bladder – the rest is reabsorbed. For a drug that is not reabsorbed, that means that the urine concentration is much larger than the plasma concentration. In fact, the C_{urine}/C_u for such a drug equals GFR/Urine flow. The urine flow is normally about 1–2 mL/min.

4.3.5 Heterogenous organs

So far we have considered organs or tissues such that the organ transfer function $H(t)$ in the relation

$$C_{out} = (H * C_{in})(t)$$

Box 4.4 An ultrashort overview of the anatomy and physiology of the kidneys

---

The functional unit of the kidneys is the *nephron*, of which there are about 10^6, all connected in parallel with each other. The transformation from plasma to urine begins at the *glomerulus*, which is a network of capillaries in the renal circulation. These capillary walls are about 50 times more permeable than those of, e.g., muscle, impermeable only to the largest molecules, like the plasma proteins. The hydrostatic pressure in the renal capillaries is about twice that of other capillaries, which is necessary in order to overcome the osmotic pressure and get a net filtration.

When fluid leaves the glomerulus it enters the proximal part of the tubule. As this glomerular filtrate passes down the tubules, its volume is reduced and its composition altered by the processes of tubular reabsorption (removal of water and solutes from the tubular fluid) and tubular secretion (secretion of solutes into the tubular fluid) to form urine.

About 80% of the glomerular filtrate is reabsorbed in the proximal tubules, including active reabsorption of certain substances, such as glucose. The main driving force for the reabsorption of water and electrolytes from the proximal tubules is an active transport of sodium ions, Na^+, out of the tubular lumen, which leads to a concomitant flow of chloride ions, Cl^-, and an osmotic reabsorption of water in order to keep the tubular fluid roughly isotonic with the plasma. Reabsorption depends on physiological variables like urine flow and urine acidity.

The urine is to a large extent concentrated in the next part of the nephron, an anatomical structure called the loops of Henle. A final adjustment of the urine content to body needs is done in the distal parts of the nephron, the distal tubules and collecting duct. This process is to a large extent under hormonal control. When the *antidiuretic hormone* is present water is absorbed in these parts. When it is absent the walls are impermeable to water.

---

is a mono-exponential function. In such an organ the drug is well mixed and its concentration is described by equation 4.8. For some drugs and tissues, $H(t)$ may have more phases, indicating that there are internal barriers which the drug has to overcome in order to be distributed within the tissue. A simple model of a tissue consists of an interstitial compartment and an intracellular compartment, separated by cell membranes. This gives us three concentrations to consider: the arterial concentration C_{in}, the concentration in the interstitial fluid, C_{is}, and the intracellular concentration, C_{ic}.

The most important driver for exchange of substance over membranes is diffusion. Diffusion is the natural tendency for molecules to find space for themselves. This means that the net flux of these molecules is down the concentration gradient and with a magnitude given by

$$\text{rate of penetration} = P\Delta C.$$

Here the proportionality constant P, the diffusion coefficient, is the product of a drug specific permeability coefficient and the membrane area. Hydrophilic molecules cannot pass readily through the double lipid-layer of the cell membrane but membranes contain micro-pores through which such molecules can pass. Their diffusion coefficient P is therefore small. Micro-pores are not necessary for the passage of lipid soluble molecules, including oxygen and carbon-dioxide, so such molecules have much larger diffusion coefficients. Diffusion continues until equilibrium is achieved, at which time the concentration is the same in the aqueous phases on both sides of the membrane (movement continues thereafter as well, but the net flux is zero). The time to equilibrium is determined by the diffusion constant P.

At the border between blood and a tissue, the blood flow causes a concentration gradient. When P is large, like for lipid substances, the equilibrium may be virtually instantaneous, so that the rate-limiting step that controls absorption of the drug into the cells is the blood flow. We then talk about perfusion limited absorption into the organ. Other drugs, with low P, are relatively insensitive to changes in perfusion – the problem now lies in penetrating the membrane. At low blood flows there may be enough time to penetrate a membrane, but at higher flows there is not sufficient time and the absorption then becomes independent of blood flow, giving us a permeability limited absorption into the organ.

When writing down what happens to a drug within the interstitial space of an organ we have to take into account diffusion over both the vascular wall and the cell membranes of the tissue cells and that it is the free drug that penetrates membranes. To this we need to add what may come from filtration and subtract the amount per time unit which is transported away by the lymph system. We do not write down this equation, but instead the equation for the intracellular concentration of drug, in the case of an eliminating organ, for instance, the liver. Since it is free drug that diffuses and the intrinsic clearance is defined relative to free drug, this equation becomes

$$V_{ic}C'_{ic} = P(C_{u,is} - C_{u,ic}) - CL_{int}C_{u,ic},$$

where $C_{u,ic}$ is the free concentration within the cell and $C_{u,is}$ is the concentration of free drug in the interstitial fluid. P is the diffusion coefficient for movement over the cell membrane. At steady state, when the left hand side is zero, we find that

$$C_{u,ic} = \rho C_{u,is}, \quad \text{where } \rho = \frac{P}{P + CL_{int}}.$$

So, if we determine clearance *in vitro* looking at enzyme reactions, to get the correct extraction ratio *in vivo* we have to replace CL_{int} by ρCL_{int}, where

CL_{int} is the *in vitro* clearance. This is valid at least if free drug in the interstitial space is in rapid equilibrium with that in the blood.

4.4 Building a physiological PK model

In this section, we are going to take a look at how we can build a physiological pharmacokinetic model. Such a model can be useful for many purposes. If we have built such a model for a particular drug, we can vary the physiological parameters to see what effects exercise, or a specific disease, can have on plasma concentrations. We will not make this exercise here. Instead our objective is to build a model that reflects some key features of body physiology, and then see how the non-compartmental analysis of Chapter 2 describes this model in terms of standard pharmacokinetic concepts. The model will be a perfusion limited model and is therefore defined in terms of blood flow, organ volumes, and partition coefficients, and consequently similar to a recirculation model that was discussed in Section 2.6. The NCA analysis turns that into a volume/clearance based description which we will try to link to its model origin.

4.4.1 A recirculation model

Before we describe the specific physiological model, which is to be perfusion limited, we will make a more general discussion on how to connect individual organs described by transfer functions into groups of organs and finally a whole body.

First, assume that we have the situation of Figure 4.2(a) with two organs in parallel. We want to determine the transfer function $H(t)$ for the pair of organs. We have $Q = Q_1 + Q_2$, and organ i has transfer function $H_i(t)$. In this situation we have

$$QC_{out}(t) = Q_1C_1(t) + Q_2C_2(t) = Q_1(H_1 * C_{in})(t) + Q_2(H_2 * C_{in})(t),$$

so we see that

$$H(t) = \frac{Q_1}{Q}H_1(t) + \frac{Q_2}{Q}H_2(t).$$

It follows directly that (with E_i the extraction ratio of organ i)

$$I(H) = \frac{Q_1}{Q}(1 - E_1) + \frac{Q_2}{Q}(1 - E_2), \quad E(H) = \frac{Q_1}{Q}E(H_1) + \frac{Q_2}{Q}E(H_2),$$

from which we deduce that the mean transit time over the pair of organs is a weighted sum of the mean transit times of the individual organs:

$$MTT(H) = \frac{Q_1(1 - E_1)MTT(H_1) + Q_2(1 - E_2)MTT(H_2)}{Q_1(1 - E_1) + Q_2(1 - E_2)}.$$

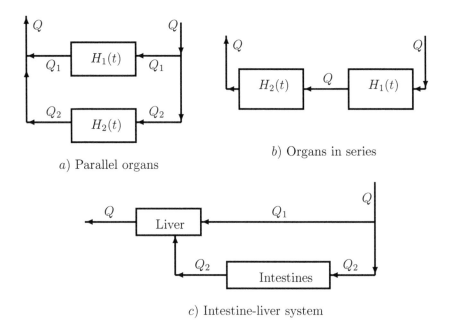

a) Parallel organs

b) Organs in series

c) Intestine-liver system

FIGURE 4.2: Elementary organ connections

Next we consider two organs in series; see Figure 4.2(b). Now the flow is the same over each organ and we have $C_1 = H_1 * C_{in}$ and $C_{out} = H_2 * C_1$. So it follows that $H = H_2 * H_1$ and consequently

$$\mathrm{MTT}(H) = \mathrm{MTT}(H_1) + \mathrm{MTT}(H_2).$$

Other examples can be built from this. For example, the intestines-liver system shown in Figure 4.2(c) can be considered built up of two parallel organs, one consisting of a part of the liver alone, the other of the rest of the liver and the intestines. A derivation of the transfer function for the system from first principles is that

$$QC_{out} = H_1 * (Q_1 C_a) + H_1 * (Q_2 C_2) = (Q_1 H_1 + Q_2(H_1 * H_2)) * C_{in},$$

so the total transfer function is

$$H(t) = \frac{Q_1}{Q} H_1(t) + \frac{Q_2}{Q}(H_1 * H_2)(t).$$

A short computation then shows that

$$\mathrm{MTT}(H) = \mathrm{MTT}(H_1) + \frac{Q_2(1 - E_2)\mathrm{MTT}(H_2)}{Q - Q_2 E_2}.$$

We will now consider a simplification of the circulatory system of the human body, consisting only of the organs listed in Table 4.1 and with the data given in that table. What this model body looks like is graphically illustrated in Figure 4.3, where percentages of cardiac output are given to the right in the figure and organ volumes to the left.

A careful look at Figure 4.3 shows that the circulatory system consists of two parts lying in series. Part I consists of the veins, lungs, and arteries and Part II of the other organs, most of which lie in parallel connecting the arteries with the veins. The organs in Part I all lie in series, so its transfer function is given by

$$H_I(t) = (H_{veins} * H_{lungs} * H_{arteries})(t).$$

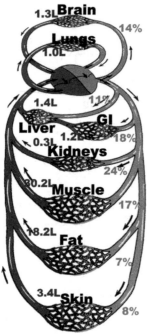

For Part II we have six organs in parallel, if we consider the intestines and liver as one organ:

$$H_{II}(t) = \sum_i \frac{Q_i}{Q_c} H_i(t).$$

The function $H = H_I * H_{II}$ then has the property

$$Q_c C_a = H * (Q_c C_a),$$

and describes the one-pass circulation of a drug molecule. $H(t)$ is therefore similar to the function describing drug circulation in the recirculation model in Section 2.6.

We do not write out an explicit expression for the function $H(t)$ for this simplified model of the body, though it can be deduced from the formulas above. Instead we restrict ourselves to an expression for the mean drug circulation time, which we do under the assumption that all elimination occurs in the liver.

FIGURE 4.3: The vascular system of a simplified human body

From the discussion above we have that

$$t_{circ} = \mathrm{MTT}(H_I) + \mathrm{MTT}(H_{II}),$$

and that

$$\mathrm{MTT}(H_I) = \sum_{i \in \mathcal{I}} \mathrm{MTT}(H_i),$$

where the index set $\mathcal{I}$ consists of the veins, lungs, and arteries.

For Part II we have, if the index set $\mathcal{I}$ now contains all organs in the systemic circulation except the intestines and the liver, that

$$Q_c E(H_{II}) = \sum_{i \in \mathcal{I}} Q_i \text{MTT}(H_i) + Q_l(1 - E)\text{MTT}(H_s),$$

where H_s is the transfer function for the intestines-liver system and Q_l the liver blood flow. Note that all organs in $\mathcal{I}$ are assumed non-eliminating. But $(l = \text{liver})$

$$\text{MTT}(H_s) = \text{MTT}(H_l) + \frac{Q_{GI}}{Q_l}\text{MTT}(H_{GI})$$

and $I(H_s) = I(H_l) = 1 - E$, so

$$Q_c I(H_{II}) = \sum_{i \in \mathcal{I}} Q_i + Q_l(1 - E) = Q_c - EQ_l.$$

It follows that $(Q_c - EQ_l)\text{MTT}_{II}$ equals

$$\sum_i Q_i\text{MTT}(H_i) - E(Q_l\text{MTT}(H_l) + Q_{GI}\text{MTT}(H_{GI})).$$

From this we can deduce a formula for overall circulation time t_{circ} as an appropriately weighted sum of organ transit times.

We have called the model just described a recirculation model, but strictly speaking it is not. It is a Markov state model, with states consisting of the different tissues. A drug molecule stays in a particular state for a duration of time described by the transfer function of the state/tissue. Transitions between states are governed by the circuit schema of Figure 4.3, with probabilities being ratios of flows. This means that it is not the flow at a particular point in the circulation system that can be our measurement, but the content of one of the organs. If we measure in the veins, the recirculation model we get is

$$M_v(t) = F(t) + (H * M_v)(t). \tag{4.9}$$

Here $M_v(t)$ is the amount of drug in the veins at time t, $H(t)$ the transfer function of the body and $F(t)$ the amount of drug that is in the veins for the first time at time t. If we apply a bolus dose to the veins, this means that $F(t)$ is the amount of dose that has not left the veins at time t.

4.4.2 Physiological perfusion limited models

In this section we will specialize our model assumptions one step further and build a perfusion limited physiological pharmacokinetics model. This means that we assume all tissues to be one-compartmental, i.e., well mixed with a well-defined concentration. Our example will be based on the same

assumption as in the previous paragraph, i.e., the prototype human illustrated in Figure 4.3.The arguments allow for larger models with more tissues
connected in more complicated networks. We will model a drug that is eliminated by metabolism in the liver only and by an enzyme system that is in
such abundance that we can assume the intrinsic clearance to be constant.

The model consists of a system of differential equations built up from equations 4.5 and 4.6, except that we will formulate it in terms of the concentrations $C_i(t)$ of drug leaving the organ i, so that $C_i(t) = C_T(t)/K_{p,i}$, if $C_T(t)$
is the concentration in that tissue. It is convenient to give the concentrations
in arterial and venous blood the notations $C_a(t), C_v(t)$ respectively.

For a non-eliminating organ we now have that

$$V_i K_{p,i} C_i'(t) = Q_i(C_a(t) - C_i(t)),$$

provided the concentration in all ingoing vessels is the arterial concentration.
This is not the case for the lungs, where the ingoing concentration should be
$C_v(t)$ instead. For the only eliminating organ, the liver, the equation becomes
(cf Figure 4.2(c))

$$V_i K_{p,i} C_i'(t) = Q_1(C_a(t) - C_i(t)) + Q_2(C_{GI}(t) - C_i(t)) - CL_{int}' C_i(t).$$

Here Q_1 represents the flow of the hepatic artery, which carries drug of concentration $C_a(t)$, whereas Q_2 is the flow of the portal vein, which carries blood
from the gastrointestinal tract with concentration $C_{GI}(t)$, which in turn is one
of the C_i's above. CL_{int}' is the intrinsic clearance times the fraction unbound
drug in the liver.

There are two organs yet not considered, the veins and the arteries. The
equation for the former is

$$V_v C_v'(t) = \sum_{i \in \mathcal{I}} Q_i C_i(t) - Q_c C_v(t),$$

where Q_c is the cardiac output and $\mathcal{I}$ is a list of all the organs that feed
into the venous circulation (note that $Q_c = \sum_{i \in \mathcal{I}} Q_i$). The equation for the
arteries is

$$V_a C_a'(t) = Q_c(C_{lungs}(t) - C_a(t)).$$

We can now administer drug to this system anywhere we want to. We
can, for instance, add a tablet that is absorbed from the intestines, or we can
administer a drug intra-vascularly. A bolus dose given intravenously can be
modelled by assuming $C_v(0) = D/V_v$ with all other start concentrations zero.

The parameters of this system of equations are divided into those that are
body specific (the tissue volumes and blood flows) and those that are drug
specific (the partition coefficients). The latter need to be determined for each
drug, and are generally assumed to be the same for all species, and therefore
estimated in some particular animal species.

Example 4.4

The physiological model we are going to discuss assumes a bolus dose administration into the veins of the prototype human body in Figure 4.3. The physiological data is that given in Table 4.1 and we use the following partition coefficients (completely arbitrarily chosen)

Organ: Liver Kidneys GI tract Lungs Brain Muscles Adipose tissue Skin
K_p: 2.6   1.3   4.1   1.0   1.6   2.1   5.0   1.0

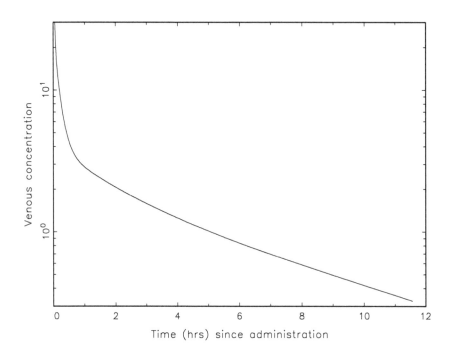

FIGURE 4.4: Predicted venous blood concentrations from perfusion model

We assume that CL'_{int} equals 1500 mL/min, which corresponds to a hepatic extraction ratio of 0.51. For this model, which results in a system of differential equations as described above, we can compute the solution, for which the venous concentration curve is shown in Figure 4.4.

The amount of drug in organ i at time t is given by $V_i K_{p,i} C_i(t)$. From that we can first compute the total amount of drug in the body at time t as

$$M(t) = V_a C_a(t) + V_v C_v(t) + \sum_i V_i K_{p,i} C_i(t).$$

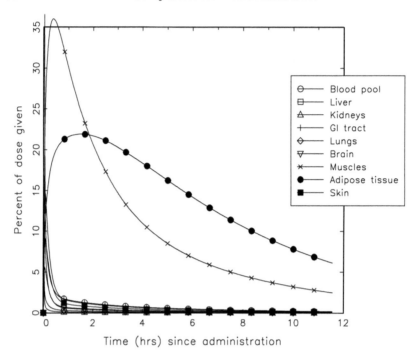

FIGURE 4.5: Predicted amount drug in each organ from perfusion model

The amounts, as percent of given dose, in individual tissues at different times are shown in Figure 4.5. It illustrates how the change in amount in the tissues depends on the tissue rate constants $k_T = Q/V_T K_p$: we see that drug is absorbed into, and therefore eliminated from, muscle and adipose tissue much more slowly than other tissues as the following table of tissue rate constants confirms

Liver	Kidneys	GI tract	Lungs	Brain	Muscles	Adipose tissue	Skin
0.40	3.3	0.18	5.6	0.32	0.017	0.0051	0.15

We see that the limiting factor for elimination from the body lies in the reserves that are built up in the adipose tissue and muscles. Drugs are released by these organs much more slowly than the true elimination rate in the liver. In fact, it is impossible to distinguish the other curves from each other in Figure 4.5, indicating that a simpler model in which all these tissues are lumped together into one organ would be difficult to distinguish from the present model. We will take that discussion up in Chapter 5.

From this we now compute the distribution volume, which is defined by $V(t) = M(t)/C_v(t)$ since we measure at a venous site. It is shown as the solid curve in Figure 4.6, which has a steep increase during the first hour to 200 liters, and then a further slower increase to an asymptotic value of 283 liters. In passing we note that

$$V_{ss} = V_a + V_v + \sum_i V_i K_{p,i} = 175 \text{ liters,}$$

and that, using the formula on pages 84–85, we can also calculate the circulation time to 37 minutes.

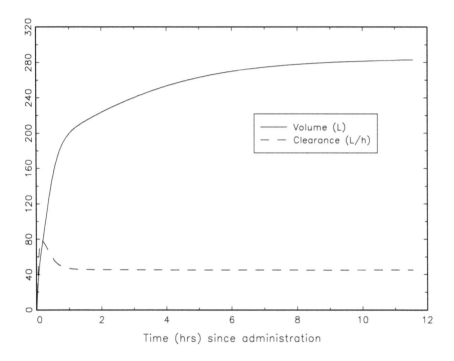

FIGURE 4.6: The apparent volume $V(t)$ and clearance function $CL(t)$ under the perfusion model

Figure 4.6 also contains a description of the clearance function. To compute clearance, we observe that the rate of elimination at time t is given by $CL'_{int}C_{liver}(t)$, so the clearance function is

$$CL(t) = CL'_{int}C_{liver}(t)/C_v(t).$$

As we see in Figure 4.6 this is time-dependent during the first half hour or so. This is because elimination does not occur from the compartment we measure in, in the veins, but in the liver. To be eliminated the drug first has to leave the blood and enter the liver, which gives this transient behavior. Soon, however, as blood and liver equilibrate, it settles down to a value of about 45 L/h, or 749 mL/min.

With reference to Figure 4.6 we see that if we assume a constant clearance (relative to venous blood) we should not be too much in error.   □

The model we constructed in Example 4.4 is a compartment model with ten compartments. It tries to capture some key anatomical and physiological aspects of how very lipophilic substances may be transported around the body. Our standard model for pharmacokinetic analysis, the non-compartmental approach to analysis, ignores most of what this model is built upon: blood flows, perfusion ratios etc. It is therefore of interest to make a NCA analysis of the venous plasma concentration curve and see how the PK parameters one derives from it relates to the ones of the model.

We will do this not from the true, continuous data, but from a sample of data. And we will not sample at time zero. This will force us to reconstruct $C_v(0)$ by backward extrapolation from the samples taken. We will assume exact plasma concentrations whenever measured – no assay problems at all.

Example 4.5
We will now do a non-compartmental analysis of the venous blood concentration curve in Figure 4.4. We assume that we sample at times 1, 2, 5 and 10 minutes, and then every tenth minute up to and including 690 minutes after start (unrealistically rich number of samples). To obtain a sample at time $t = 0$ we extrapolate log-linearly backwards, using the first two observed points. The NCA analysis produces the following list of standard PK parameters:

$t_{1/2}$ (h)	CL (mL/min)	MRT (h)	V_c (L)	V_{ss} (L)	V_d (L)
4.3	756	3.9	6.8	177	282

Note that V_c is larger than the true starting volume. The reason for this is precisely that we did not sample at time zero, and therefore allowed recirculation to occur before we get any data points. The initial dose, which was confined to the venous site, was during the first minute distributed over the total blood volume and more. The definition of V_c rests on blood/plasma and everything in rapid equilibrium with it. That is a rather imprecise definition, since it will depend on our exact time points of measurement, as this example shows.

In fact, we can identify what the analysis picks up as the central compartment. Inspecting the tissue rate constants we find that two of them are > 1, those for kidneys and lungs. Also the volume $V_a + V_v + V_{lungs} + K_{kidneys} V_{kidneys}$ agrees with the central volume V_c estimate. So the NCA analysis has identified these four organs as in rapid diffusive equilibrium with a common drug concentration.

The estimates of the other volumes of the standard model for pharmacokinetic analysis, volume in steady state and volume of distribution, agree well with their "true" values; e.g., V_d is in good agreement with what we see in Figure 4.6. Also V_{ss} is close to the true one. Note, however, that the model is one in which we have peripheral elimination, and then the volume in steady state should be underestimated. This is because it is based on MRT_{app}, which has to be smaller than the true MRT, since information in plasma cannot capture the time spent in the liver cells before elimination. Also clearance agrees reasonably well with what we found in Figure 4.6. ▯

So the standard approach to analysis of pharmacokinetic data correctly catches the information it makes claims about. Another approach to modelling was discussed in Section 2.6, which was based on a circulatory system. In the next example we analyze our data from that perspective, using equation 4.9.

Example 4.6
We now want to analyze the same data under the model defined by equation 4.9. Since we have put the amount D in the vein, the function describing the amount that is in the veins for the first time is given by $F(t) = De^{-k_v t}$, where k_v is the tissue rate for veins, about 1.6 per hour. It is therefore almost zero within minutes, and we solve the equation $C_v(t) = H * C_v(t)$ for $t \geq 10$ minutes only. This analysis is very sensitive to details in drug concentrations at the start, and in order to get agreement with true numbers we, for this analysis only, choose to use the true $C_v(0)$ when computing the integral in equation 4.9. We will discuss this point further in Section 5.6.

Figure 4.7 shows the one-pass circulation function $H(t)$, obtained by numerical deconvolution, and from it we can estimate the whole body extraction ratio to 0.13. This agrees with the liver extraction ratio of the previous section, since the liver flow for this model is 27% of the cardiac output. The circulation time t_{circ} is estimated to 34 minutes, which implies an estimate of MRT to 3.8 hours. All numbers are in reasonable agreement with the true values, computed in example 4.4, and the values obtained in the NCA analysis in example 4.5. ▯

4.5   Absorption from the intestines

When we ingest a solution of a drug, the mechanism for absorption of the active ingredient is essentially not different from that accounting for drug distribution in the body. The drug needs to pass through the intestinal wall in order to be taken up by the blood. The driving force for this uptake is the difference in concentrations between the solution in the intestines, denoted

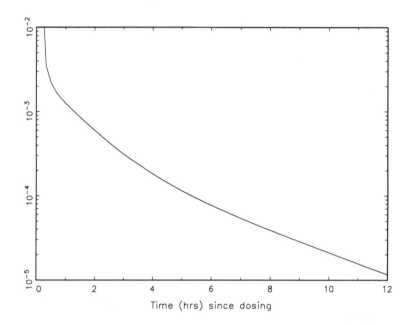

Time (hrs) since dosing

FIGURE 4.7: The function $H(t)$ of recirculation time

C_s, and the unbound concentration in blood. During this absorption process we therefore have the same kind of barriers as for any distributional process, including both permeability limited and perfusion limited absorption, or a combination of these.

If the plasma concentration of free drug is negligible compared to the intestinal concentration, this means that the uptake rate of drug should be of the form $P(C_s - C_u) \approx PC_s$, where P is the diffusion coefficient (as before, the product of a permeability constant and the surface area over which absorption takes place). One extreme occurs when the concentration in the intestines is kept (virtually) constant, so that the amount that is taken up per time unit is constant. This is zero order absorption, and it is, mathematically, equivalent to a constant rate infusion. The other extreme is when the drug is dissolved in a fixed volume, V_a, with varying concentration. Then the rate of absorption is $k_a M(t)$, where $M(t)$ is the amount in the intestines and $k_a = P/V_a$. Thus the absorption is first order and we have that $M'(t) = -k_a M(t)$ if there is no other loss of drug than to the blood stream.

Often there are good reasons not to administer a drug as a solution, but instead to give it in a solid form. Tablets and capsules are the most important examples. How, and to what extent, such solids are absorbed turns out to depend also on the manufacture processes. For this reason we can never assume that a new formulation automatically will produce a tablet that has the same effects as the original tablet, even if the dose is the same. Consequently a change in formulation or manufacture process requires an investigation of the absorption process in a bioequivalence study.

The process that leads to a solid drug formulation being absorbed into the blood stream has two distinct steps:

$$\text{solid drug} \longrightarrow \text{drug in solution} \longrightarrow \text{absorbed drug.}$$

Note that any of these two steps can be rate-limiting. If it is the second step that is rate-limiting, there will be more drug in solution in the intestines than if it is the dissolution that is rate-limiting. The mean absorption time, as defined earlier, is the time it takes from the drug is swallowed until it appears in plasma, and should therefore be split up as the sum of the Mean Dissolution Time (MDT) and the true Mean Absorption Time. It would therefore be appropriate to rename our original definition of MAT as the Mean Time at the Input Site, but since this discussion is not prolonged beyond this section, we will not do that.

To describe the dissolution of a solid, let $M(t)$ be the amount of undissolved drug in the intestines at time t. Assume that the dissolution rate is proportional to the concentration difference $C_s - C(t)$ between the concentration of drug in the saturated solution at the surface of the solid, C_s, and the concentration of the drug in the dissolution media, the intestinal juice, at time t, $C(t)$. Thus, in analogy with above,

$$M'(t) = -kA(t)(C_s - C(t)),$$

where k is some constant and $A(t)$ the total surface area at time t of the solid. Assuming that dissolution changes the dimensions of the tablet, but not its shape, we can assume that $A(t)$ is proportional to $M(t)^b$ for $b = 2/3$.

To this is added the complication that comes from the anatomy and physiology of the gastro-intestinal tract. Usually drug is absorbed in the intestines and not in the stomach. Dissolution may, however, occur in the stomach. This means that drug absorption will not commence until there has been a gastric emptying, which may take time. For a drug that needs the acid environment of the stomach for proper dissolution, the time spent in the stomach will be an important determinant of how much drug can eventually be absorbed, since it determines how much of the drug will turn into a form that can be absorbed. Also, the speed with which drug is transported through the intestines is important for how much drug that is actually taken up by the body.

4.6 Chapter epilogue: An alternative liver model

The well mixed organ model discussed above was as follows: each organ is considered to be an aqueous container of a certain volume V_T in which all drug that enters is instantly and completely mixed into a concentration C_T. Drug is presented to the organ by an amount QC_{in} per time unit. On the output side, free drug is in instant equilibrium with what is in the outgoing vessel and protein binding is also an instantaneous process, so that the concentration in that vessel is given by $C_{out} = C_T/K_p$ where K_p is the partition coefficient.

This model is perhaps not in complete agreement with the anatomical arrangement of how blood flows in a tissue. Anatomically, capillaries penetrate the organ as small tubes, and it is across their walls drug exchange occur. In doing so we expect the drug concentration in the capillaries to change smoothly along the capillaries, from the entry concentration C_{in} to the output concentration C_{out}. We will now discuss a simple model that takes this into account, and see how that relates to the simpler well-stirred model discussed in this chapter.

The model is called the parallel tube model of the liver, and assumes that the ingoing vessel to the liver splits up into a large number of identical parallel vessels which then fuse into one outgoing vessel. This model will also assume that free drug in the capillary is in instant equilibrium with what is in the tissue, only that now this is true along the whole capillary. We consider a capillary of length L and constant cross-sectional area A, and denote the concentration at the point x as $C(t, x)$. As boundary conditions we have

$$C(t, 0) = C_{in}(t), \qquad C(t, L) = C_{out}(t).$$

Since we have instant equilibrium of free drug between blood and tissue, we can assume that the removal of drug actually occurs within the blood. If the intrinsic clearance CL_{int} is assumed constant along the whole capillary and the removal is evenly spread along it, the intrinsic clearance that operates on the concentration $C(t, x)$ is CL_{int}/L. We can now derive a mass-balance equation by considering a piece V_x of the capillary starting at the point x and with width Δx and cross-sectional area A. Let Q be the capillary flow. Mass-balance tells us that the rate of change of amount of drug in V_x is the net flow of drug over its boundaries minus what is eliminated:

$$\frac{\partial}{\partial t} \int_{V_x} C(t, y) dy = QAC(t, x) - QAC(t, x + \Delta x) - \frac{f_u CL_{int}}{L} \int_{V_x} C(t, y) dy.$$

If we use that the volume of V_x is $A\Delta x$ we have that

$$QAC(t, x + \Delta x) - QAC(t, x) = Q \int_{V_x} \frac{\partial C}{\partial y}(t, y) dy,$$

so if we let V_x shrink to the point x we arrive at the partial differential equation

$$\frac{\partial C}{\partial t}(t, x) = -Q \frac{\partial C}{\partial x}(t, x) - CL_{int} f_u C(t, x)/L. \tag{4.10}$$

From this we find that the equilibrium concentrations $C(x)$ should satisfy

$$-QC'(x) = CL_{int} f_u C(x)/L,$$

which we can integrate to obtain

$$C(x) = C_{in}e^{-f_u CL_{int}x/LQ},$$

and consequently we must have

$$C_{out} = C_{in}e^{-f_u CL_{int}/Q}.$$

It follows that the extraction ratio for this tubular model is given by

$$E = \frac{C_{in} - C_{out}}{C_{in}} = 1 - e^{-f_u CL_{int}/Q}.$$

We see that like for the well mixed model, the extraction ratio is a function of $x = f_u CL_{int}/Q$. For the well-mixed model this function is $x/(1+x)$, whereas for the tubular model it is $1 - e^{-x}$. To appreciate the difference between these results, we can note that for the well-mixed model we have an extraction ratio of 0.5 if $x = 1$, whereas the corresponding value for the tubular model is $x = \ln(2) \approx 0.7$.

The fact that the relationship between extraction ratio and x is different for the two models is mainly important in the situation where we want to use an observed extraction ratio to compute the intrinsic clearance of a drug that is metabolized in the liver.

Chapter 5

Modelling the distribution process

5.1 The peripheral space

In this chapter we will discuss some approaches to modelling the distribution process of a drug. In Chapter 4 we have discussed some of the factors, including drug properties like its size and how lipophil or soluble the drug is, that influence how a particular drug becomes distributed in the body. In this chapter we leave the physiological background aside but want to find ways to describe the distribution of a given drug in the body, based on only the information that is given by its plasma profile. We want descriptions that give us additional information to the basic volume description of Chapter 2.

As before we define the central compartment as the part of the body that contains the sampling space or is in rapid equilibrium with it. This is the space over which a bolus dose instantaneously distributes itself, giving us a starting concentration. As before, the volume of the central space is denoted V_c.

Starting from this, there are two options. Either the well-mixed drug in the central compartment makes up all drug in the body, or it does not. In the latter case we define the *peripheral space* as everything else, i.e., the total body space the drug is distributed in minus the central compartment. Between the central compartment and the peripheral space there is a slower exchange of drug molecules. It is important to note that we make no assumption at this stage about the structure of the peripheral space; it may be homogenous, it may not. In fact, it may not even consist only of physical space, but can also contain biochemical transformations of the drug as discussed in Section 5.2.4.

Notation-wise we let $M_c(t)$ be the amount of drug in the central space at time t, and $M_p(t)$ the amount of drug in the peripheral space at time t, so that $M(t) = M_c(t) + M_p(t)$. As usual, let $C(t)$ be the concentration in the central compartment and V_c its volume, so that $M_c(t) = V_c C(t)$. As before when we discuss distribution and elimination, we assume that we have given a bolus dose D. Expressed in words, mass-balance considerations then produce the following two equations.

$$M'_c(t) = \quad \{\text{flow from peripheral to central space}\} -$$
$$\{\text{flow from central to peripheral space}\} -$$
$$\{\text{elimination flow from central space}\}$$
$$M'_p(t) = \quad \{\text{flow from central to peripheral space}\} -$$
$$\{\text{flow peripheral to central space}\} -$$
$$\{\text{elimination flow from peripheral space}\}$$

In this chapter we will build models by making more or less specific assumptions on the terms in the right hand sides of these two equations.

Processes in the central compartment should be proportional to the concentration of drug in the central compartment. We therefore first assume that the outward flow from the central to the peripheral compartment can be written as

$$\{\text{flow from central to peripheral space}\} = CL_d C(t).$$

The factor CL_d is called the *distributional clearance*. Similarly, we define the central (elimination) clearance CL_c by

$$\{\text{elimination flow from central space}\} = CL_c C(t).$$

These two factors can in general be allowed to be functions of time, possibly via $C(t)$. We can, for instance, assume a capacity limited elimination rate as in Section 2.5, or we can assume that the transfer from central to peripheral space is an active process and therefore also capacity limited. In our development in this chapter, we will always assume that CL_d is constant, whereas $CL_c(t)$ may be held general, allowing for capacity limited elimination from the central compartment. It follows that the first equation above will take the form

$$V_c C'(t) = \{\text{flow from peripheral to central space}\} - (CL_d + CL_c(t))C(t).$$

In Section 5.2 we will look at the situation when also the peripheral space is a compartment. In such a situation, the differential equations for $M_c(t)$ and $M_p(t)$ become a linear 2×2-system (equations 5.4 and 5.5 below) with constant coefficients which are rate constants describing the flow between the two compartments and out of the body. After having derived the standard PK parameters of Chapter 2 in terms of these rate constants, we will see that this model can be re-written as the single equation

$$V_c C'(t) = (h * C)(t) - (CL_d + CL_c(t))C(t), \tag{5.1}$$

where $h(t)$ is a mono-exponential function describing transfer through the peripheral compartment, at least if there is no elimination from the peripheral compartment. If there is peripheral elimination, the situation will turn out to be slightly more complicated.

In Section 5.3 we will go to the next level of complexity, in which we assume that the peripheral space is made up of two disjoint compartments. More precisely, we will study three-compartment models which are given as a linear 3×3-system of differential equations with constant coefficients for the amount in each compartment. The immediate problem is that since we only have data from the central space, there are too many unknown rate constants in the model compared to what we can estimate. How this problem may be handled is discussed in a few examples before we note that also in this case we can write the equation for the central compartment, assuming central elimination, as equation 5.1, but now $h(t)$ is a bi-exponential function.

With more compartments, the identification problem encountered for three-compartment models only grows. We will not discuss any such models, but note that extending the argument that derived equation 5.1 for three-compartment models, it is easy to see that a q-compartment model will give us the same equation for the central compartment (assuming central elimination) with $h(t)$ now a $q - 1$-exponential function. For that reason we take this equation as our starting point in Section 5.4 when we take a general approach to the problem of describing the distribution of a drug. Since concentration in the central compartment are the data we have, the identification of $h(t)$ is precisely the information we have on distributional aspects of the drug. We therefore discuss in some detail both some new PK parameters that describe distribution and are derived from $h(t)$, and how to estimate $h(t)$ from the available data.

In this chapter there will be much discussion on the effect of peripheral elimination of the drug. This may not be a common situation in real life, but from the viewpoint of a mathematical treatise of pharmacokinetics it is natural not to restrict the discussion to the simpler case of only central elimination of drug.

5.2   Two-compartment models

5.2.1   The two-compartment model parameters in rate constants

A two-compartment model is a model in which the peripheral space is assumed to be homogenous, so that the drug is well mixed within it, and the exchange rates between the two compartments, as well as elimination, are constants. In this section we therefore assume that both CL_d and CL_c are constants.

Let V_p be the volume of the peripheral compartment, and $C_p(t)$ its concentration at time t, so that $M_p(t) = V_p C_p(t)$. These are usually not observable (for an exception, see Section 5.2.4), but they allow us to introduce of two further flow constants, analogous to above:

$$\{\text{flow from peripheral to central space}\} = BC_p(t),$$

$$\{\text{elimination flow from peripheral space}\} = EC_p(t).$$

For a bolus dose into the central compartment, we can summarize this in the following two equations:

$$V_c C'(t) = BC_p(t) - CL_d C(t) - CL_c C(t), \quad C(0) = D/V_c \qquad (5.2)$$
$$V_p C'_p(t) = CL_d C(t) - BC_p(t) - EC_p(t), \quad C_p(0) = 0. \qquad (5.3)$$

It is customary in compartment models to rewrite this in terms of the amount functions $M_c(t)$ and $M_p(t)$ instead:

$$M'_c(t) = k_{pc} M_p(t) - (k_{cp} + k_{ce}) M_c(t), \quad M_c(0) = D, \qquad (5.4)$$
$$M'_p(t) = k_{cp} M_c(t) - (k_{pc} + k_{pe}) M_p(t), \quad M_p(0) = 0, \qquad (5.5)$$

where

$$k_{cp} = \frac{CL_d}{V_c}, \quad k_{pc} = \frac{B}{V_p}, \quad k_{ce} = \frac{CL_c}{V_c}, \quad k_{pe} = \frac{E}{V_p},$$

all are rate constants (i.e., their unit is time^{-1}). A graphical illustration of such a model is shown in Figure 5.1.

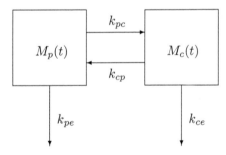

FIGURE 5.1: The two-compartment model as a model in rate constants

Note that from the rate constants we can not estimate both B, E, and the peripheral volume V_p separately, only the ratio of the former two to the latter. This is because our definition of peripheral volume and concentration is not unique: if we do not actually measure the peripheral concentration it remains unknown and we can multiply it with an arbitrary number as long as we divide V_p with the same number without changing anything else, except that B would need to be divided with the same number. This explains why only the ratios B/V_p and E/V_p are observable, not the individual components.

So far we have derived the two-compartment model equations from mass-balance considerations, without assuming a mechanistic basis for the equations. If we instead assume that the two compartments are separated by a membrane and that exchange over this membrane is by diffusion, we have that the net flow from the peripheral to the central compartment is proportional to $C_p - C$. This assumption fixes the peripheral concentration and gives us that $B = CL_d$ in equation 5.2. As discussed in Chapter 4, it is the free fraction of drug that diffuses, so there is also an implicit assumption of equal free fractions on either side of the membrane here. But assuming that, we can estimate the peripheral volume for this case as $V_p = V_c k_{cp}/k_{pc}$.

In general, however, V_p is not an observable entity, since we only make measurements in the central compartment. This is clarified somewhat if we express the volume function as

$$V(t) = \frac{M_c(t) + M_p(t)}{C(t)} = V_c + \frac{C_p(t)}{C(t)} V_p.$$

The true total volume is $V_c + V_p$, but what we measure with $V(t)$ is what the volume would have been if the concentration had been $C(t)$ throughout the body.

Note that by adding the equations 5.4 and 5.5 we find that

$$M'(t) = M_c'(t) + M_p'(t) = -k_{cp} M_c(t) - k_{pe} M_p(t).$$

Comparing this to the basic bolus equation 2.6 we obtain

$$CL(t) = CL_c + k_{pe} M_p(t)/C(t). \tag{5.6}$$

So, with only central elimination the clearance function is constant, but it is not necessarily so if there is peripheral elimination, despite the assumption that all exchange rates are constants.

5.2.2 Basic PK parameters in terms of rate constants

We are now going to compute expressions for the basic PK parameters in Table 2.1 in terms of V_c and the rate constants. These formulas are built up by $I(M_c) = V_c I(C)$ and $E(M_c) = V_c E(C)$, integrals that are obtained by applying $I(.)$ and $E(.)$ to equations 5.4 and 5.5. This gives us four linear equations in four unknowns, from which we can derive $I(M_c)$ and $E(M_c)$. From this most of the basic PK parameters can be derived. For the actual derivation, see Box 5.1. The parameters in question are

$$CL_{av} = V_c(k_{ce} + \frac{k_{cp}k_{pe}}{k_{pc} + k_{pe}}), \tag{5.7}$$

$$\text{MRT} = \frac{k_{pc} + k_{pe} + k_{cp}}{k_{ce}(k_{pc} + k_{pe}) + k_{cp}k_{pe}} \tag{5.8}$$

$$V_{ss} = CL_{av} \cdot \text{MRT} = V_c(1 + \frac{k_{cp}}{k_{pc} + k_{pe}}). \tag{5.9}$$

Another expression for MRT expresses it in the observable version, MRT_{app} (see Box 5.1):

$$\text{MRT} = \text{MRT}_{app} + \frac{k_{pe}k_{cp}}{(k_{pc} + k_{pe})(k_{ce}(k_{pc} + k_{pe}) + k_{cp}k_{pe})}, \tag{5.10}$$

where the correction term is non-zero only if there is some peripheral elimination. If we have only peripheral elimination the correction term is

$$\frac{1}{k_{pc} + k_{pe}}.$$

In the distribution process there is a point when the flow into the peripheral compartment is precisely balanced by what is eliminated from it. Such a point t_* is characterized by

$$(k_{pc} + k_{pe})M_p(t_*) = k_{cp}M_c(t_*)$$

and at such a point the volume is equal to the volume in steady state, since

$$V(t_*) = V_c + \frac{M_p(t_*)}{C(t_*)} = V_c + \frac{k_{cp}}{k_{pc} + k_{pe}}\frac{M_c(t_*)}{C(t_*)} = V_c(1 + \frac{k_{cp}}{k_{pc} + k_{pe}}) = V_{ss}.$$

There are still two basic PK parameters to derive: the terminal elimination rate and the volume of distribution. In order to express the former in terms of rate constants, we need to solve the system of equations 5.4–5.5. The theory of linear differential equations described in Section A.2 tells us that

$$M_c(t) = \frac{D}{\lambda_1 - \lambda_2}((\lambda_2 - k_{cp} - k_{ce})e^{-\lambda_1 t} + (\lambda_1 - k_{cp} - k_{ce})e^{-\lambda_2 t}), \tag{5.11}$$

$$M_p(t) = \frac{Dk_{cp}}{\lambda_1 - \lambda_2}(e^{-\lambda_2 t} - e^{-\lambda_1 t}), \tag{5.12}$$

where

$$\lambda_1, \lambda_2 = \frac{1}{2}((k_{cp} + k_{ce} + k_{pc} + k_{pe}) \pm \sqrt{(k_{cp} + k_{ce} - k_{pc} - k_{pe})^2 + 4k_{pc}k_{cp}}$$

($\lambda_2 < \lambda_1$). It is the smaller one of these which defines the terminal elimination rate λ_{el} as

$$\lambda_{el} = \frac{1}{2}(k_{cp} + k_{ce} + k_{pc} + k_{pe} - \sqrt{(k_{cp} + k_{ce} - k_{pc} - k_{pe})^2 + 4k_{pc}k_{cp}}). \tag{5.13}$$

For large t we have

$$M_c(t) \approx \frac{D}{\lambda_1 - \lambda_2}(\lambda_2 - k_{cp} - k_{ce})e^{-\lambda_2 t}, \quad M_p(t) \approx \frac{Dk_{cp}}{\lambda_1 - \lambda_2}e^{-\lambda_2 t},$$

Box 5.1 Derivation of basic PK parameters in terms of rate constants for a two-compartment model

Apply $I(.)$ and $E(.)$ to equations 5.4 and 5.5 to get the linear system

$$-D = k_{pc}I(M_p) - (k_{cp} + k_{ce})I(M_c)$$
$$0 = k_{cp}I(M_c) - (k_{pc} + k_{pe})I(M_p)$$
$$-I(M_c) = k_{pc}E(M_p) - (k_{cp} + k_{ce})E(M_c)$$
$$-I(M_p) = k_{cp}E(M_c) - (k_{pc} + k_{pe})E(M_p).$$

In order to solve this system, we first express $I(M_p)$ and $E(M_p)$ in the corresponding entities for M_c:

$$I(M_p) = XI(M_c), \quad X = \frac{k_{cp}}{k_{pc} + k_{pe}}$$

$$E(M_p) = \frac{k_{cp}E(M_c) + I(M_p)}{k_{pc} + k_{pe}} = XE(M_c) + YI(M_c), \quad Y = \frac{k_{cp}}{(k_{pc} + k_{pe})^2}.$$

The solution can be written as

$$I(M_c) = \frac{D}{k_{ce} + k_{pe}X}, \quad E(M_c) = \frac{D(1 + k_{pc}Y)}{(k_{ce} + k_{pe}X)^2}.$$

In order to derive PK parameters, we first compute the integrals

$$\int_0^\infty tCL(t)C(t)dt = k_{ce}E(M_c) + k_{pe}E(M_p) = (k_{ce} + k_{pe}X)E(M_c) + k_{pe}YI(M_c))$$

$$\int_0^\infty CL(t)C(t)dt = k_{ce}I(M_c) + k_{pe}I(M_p) = (k_{ce} + k_{pe}X)I(M_c).$$

The ratio of these gives us MRT

$$\mathrm{MRT} = \frac{E(M_c)}{I(M_c)} + \frac{k_{pe}Y}{k_{ce} + k_{pe}X}.$$

Equation 5.10 is immediate from this. Also

$$\mathrm{MRT} = \frac{1 + (k_{pc} + k_{pe})Y}{k_{ce} + k_{pe}X} = \frac{1 + X}{k_{ce} + k_{pe}X} = \frac{k_{pc} + k_{pe} + k_{cp}}{k_{ce}(k_{pc} + k_{pe}) + k_{cp}k_{pe}}.$$

Moreover,

$$CL_{av} = \frac{DV_c}{I(M_c)} = V_c(k_{ce} + k_{pe}X) = V_c(k_{ce} + \frac{k_{cp}k_{pe}}{k_{pc} + k_{pe}}),$$

and therefore $V_{ss} = CL_{av} \cdot \mathrm{MRT} =$

$$V_c(k_{ce} + k_{pe}X)\frac{1 + X}{k_{ce} + k_{pe}X} = V_c(1 + X) = V_c(1 + \frac{k_{cp}}{k_{pc} + k_{pe}}).$$

from which we deduce that

$$V(t) = V_c(1 + M_p(t)/M_c(t)) \rightarrow V_c(1 + \frac{k_{cp}}{\lambda_{el} - k_{cp} - k_{ce}}) \text{ as } t \rightarrow \infty. \quad (5.14)$$

The right hand side gives an expression for V_d in terms of V_c and rate constants, if we insert the expression for the terminal elimination rate in 5.13.

We will soon look at an example, but before we do that we want to use equation 5.11 and 5.12 and compare it to an observed equation for the central space

$$C(t) = A_1 e^{-\lambda_1 t} + A_2 e^{-\lambda_2 t},$$

in order to derive the rate constants. To do that, introduce the numbers

$$a = -k_{cp} - k_{ce}, \quad b = k_{pc}, \quad c = k_{cp}, \quad d = -k_{pc} - k_{pe}.$$

How these can be determined from $A_1, A_2, \lambda_1, \lambda_2$ is shown in Appendix A.2. With $Z = \lambda_1 - \lambda_2$ the result is that

$$a = A_2 Z V_c / D - \lambda_1, \quad d = -2\lambda_1 + Z - a, \quad bc = (Z^2 - (a - d)^2)/4. \quad (5.15)$$

Explicit formulas for how the rate constants of the compartment model are expressed in the parameters describing the plasma concentration are derived in Box 5.2. However, the example below will use equation 5.15.

Example 5.1

We revisit Example 2.1 in which a bolus dose of $D = 10$ mg gave the plasma concentration curve (mg/L)

$$C(t) = 0.38e^{-1.65t} + 0.18e^{-0.182t}.$$

We will now model this as a two-compartment model, which is possible since it is a bi-exponential function.

Referring to the last comment before the start of this example, a short calculation shows that the rate constant must satisfy

$$k_{cp} + k_{ce} = 1.18, \quad k_{pc}k_{cp} = 0.47, \quad k_{pc} + k_{pe} = 0.65.$$

This is three equations in four unknowns, so we need to make some further assumption.

Assume first that we have **central elimination** only, so that $k_{pe} = 0$. Then $k_{pc} = 0.65$, from which it follows that $k_{cp} = 0.47/0.65 = 0.72$ and from this that $k_{ce} = 1.18 - 0.72 = 0.46$. We can now deduce the two clearance terms, both with unit L/h,

$$CL_d = k_{cp}V_c = 0.72 \cdot 17.9 = 12.8, \qquad CL_c = k_{ce}V_c = 0.46 \cdot 17.9 = 8.2.$$

Box 5.2 Micro constants in terms of macro constants for a two-compartment model

---

The rate constants k_{pc}, k_{cp}, k_{ce}, and k_{pe} are often called micro constants, whereas the constants A_1, A_2, λ_1, and λ_2 defining the bi-exponential function $C(t)$ are called macro constants. We can derive an explicit relation between these two sets of constants using the relationships in equation 5.15.

First note that inserting the expression for a into the expression for d gives us

$$d = -A_2 Z V_c / D - \lambda_2.$$

From this we can deduce that

$$a - d = 2 A_2 Z V_c / D - Z,$$

which we can insert into the expression for bc to obtain

$$bc = Z^2 A_2 \frac{V_c}{D} (1 - A_2 \frac{V_c}{D}).$$

Next we observe that, since $V_c C(0) = D$,

$$V_c (A_1 + A_2) = D.$$

If we insert that into the expressions above we find that

$$k_{cp} + k_{ce} = -Z \frac{A_2}{A_1 + A_2} + \lambda_1 = \frac{\lambda_1 A_1 + \lambda_2 A_2}{A_1 + A_2},$$

$$k_{pc} + k_{pe} = -Z \frac{A_2}{A_1 + A_2} + \lambda_2 = \frac{\lambda_2 A_1 + \lambda_1 A_2}{A_1 + A_2},$$

$$k_{cp} k_{pc} = \frac{(\lambda_1 - \lambda_2)^2 A_1 A_2}{(A_1 + A_2)^2}.$$

Further reduction requires that we assume either that $k_{pe} = 0$, or that $k_{ce} = 0$, and is not discussed.

The last of these is only a verification of what we already know from the NCA in Example 2.1. In this case clearance is constant, and Figure 2.1 shows the volume curve as a function of time.

Also note a few other relationships. The terminal elimination rate λ_{el} is 0.182 per hour, whereas the true elimination rate is much larger, 0.46 per hour. This illustrates that the terminal elimination rate in the presence of distribution is the net effect of distributional changes and elimination.

If we instead assume that we have only **peripheral elimination**, i.e., that $k_{ce} = 0$, we find that $k_{cp} = 1.18$ and therefore that $CL_d = 1.18 \cdot 17.9 = 21.0$ L/h. Moreover, $k_{pc} = 0.47/1.18 = 0.40$ and $k_{pe} = 0.65 - 0.40 = 0.25$. As already noted, the clearance is now time-dependent.

Below is a table of the basic PK parameters, computed from the rate constants and V_c, in these two cases.

| | Type of elimination | |
Parameter	Central	Peripheral
CL_{av}	8.20	8.20
CL_d	12.8	21.0
MRT	4.57	6.10
V_{ss}	37.5	50.0
V_d	45.1	62.4

We see the expected consequences of peripheral elimination: larger MRT and volumes. Distributional clearance is also larger, but the elimination clearance stays the same. The parameters obtained assuming central elimination are the same as those obtained from the NCA analysis in Example 2.1.

The left plot in Figure 5.2 illustrates the inter-compartmental flows for the two cases. Solid lines represent central elimination, dashed lines peripheral elimination. Curves that start at the origin represent flow from the peripheral to the central compartments, whereas the curves that start up the y-axis represent flow from the central to the peripheral compartment. We see that the two flows intersect at the same time in both models, and that is the time that defines the volume in steady state on the volume curve.

The right plot in Figure 5.2 shows the fraction of dose given, D, that is in a particular compartment at a given time. The fraction $F_p(t) = M_p(t)/D$ that is in the peripheral room at time t is given by

$$F_p(t) = 0.68 k_{cp} (e^{-0.182t} - e^{-1.65t}).$$

Here k_{cp} is the entity that differs between central and peripheral elimination. In fact, it is $1.18/0.72 = 1.64$ times larger when we have peripheral elimination. This is natural: given what we have in plasma, there must be more drug in the peripheral space if the drug will be eliminated from it.

So far we have discussed this as a general two-compartment model. If we add the assumption that it is a diffusion driven flow, we can also estimate the peripheral volume as $V_p = CL_d/k_{pc}$. For the case with central elimination

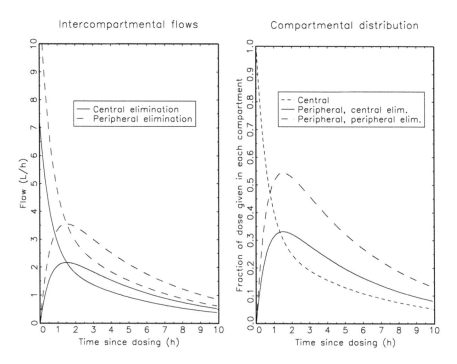

FIGURE 5.2: Illustration of inter-compartmental flows and the division of dose given between the two spaces. For explanations, see the text.

this becomes 19.6 liters, whereas if we have peripheral elimination we get 52.7 liters. Note that it is only when we have only central elimination that we have that $V_{ss} = V_c + V_p$; in the general case the relation is

$$V_{ss} = V_c + \frac{k_{pc}}{k_{pc} + k_{pe}} V_p.$$

$\square$

5.2.3 A convolution-differential equation

We can see our two-compartment model as consisting of two things: the basic concentration function $C(t)$ in a central space of constant volume V_c, and the amount in the peripheral space given by the function $M_p(t)$. There is a re-formulation of this in terms of another function which instead relates to transit time in the peripheral compartment.

In fact, we can solve Equation 5.5 for $M_p(t)$:

$$M_p(t) = k_{cp} \int_0^t e^{-(k_{pc}+k_{pe})(t-s)} M_c(s) \, ds.$$

Therefore, by introducing the function

$$h(t) = k_{cp} k_{pc} e^{-(k_{pc}+k_{pe})t},$$

we can write the flow from peripheral to central compartment as a convolution

$$k_{pc} M_p(t) = (h * M_c)(t).$$

Equation 5.4 can now be rewritten as

$$M_c'(t) = (h * M_c)(t) - (k_{cp} + k_{ce}) M_c(t), \quad M_c(0) = D.$$

The function $h(t)$ is called the transfer function for the peripheral compartment.

To understand $h(t)$, assume first that we have only central elimination. Assume that at time $t = 0$ we have M_0 units of drug in the central compartment and let Δt be a very short time interval. The amount per time unit that enters the peripheral space in that time space is then $k_{cp} M_0 \Delta t$. This amount will return to the central space spread over time: at time t the flow returning is $h(t) M_0 \Delta t$. The amount that has returned up to time t is then given by

$$M_0 \Delta t \int_0^t h(s) \, ds = k_{cp} M_0 \Delta t (1 - e^{-k_{pc}t}).$$

It follows that

$$\int_0^\infty h(t) \, dt = k_{cp},$$

and that the time a drug molecule will spend in the peripheral compartment (its transit time) is given by the distribution which has the probability function

$$\frac{h(t)}{k_{cp}} = k_{pc} e^{-k_{pc}t},$$

i.e., the exponential distribution with mean $1/k_{pc}$.

When there is peripheral elimination, the situation becomes more complicated because a drug that enters the peripheral space has two possible exit ways: to the central space and by elimination. But we can note that

$$CL(t) = CL_c + k_{pe} M_p(t)/C(t) = CL_c + V_c(e * C)(t)/C(t),$$

where

$$e(t) = k_{pe} h(t)/k_{pc} = k_{cp} k_{pe} e^{-(k_{pc}+k_{pe})t}.$$

Making some redefinitions and rearrangements, we see that the two-compartment model is in fact equivalent to the two equations

$$V_c C'(t) = (h * C)(t) - (CL_d + CL_c)C(t), \quad C(0) = D/V_c.$$

$$CL(t) = CL_c + (e * C)(t)/C(t),$$

where

$$h(t) = CL_d k_{pc} e^{-(k_{pc} + k_{pe})t}, \quad e(t) = k_{pe} h(t)/k_{pc}.$$

This idea will be generalized in Section 5.4 to the case when the peripheral space is not assumed homogenous.

5.2.4 Reversible metabolic conversion

Consider an one-compartment drug, called the parent drug, for which we have the amount $M(t)$ at time t in the body. Assume that it is metabolized, but that for one of the metabolites, this reaction is *reversible*. We assume that also the metabolite is an one-compartmental substance and denote the amount at time t in the body by $M_m(t)$. This defines a two-compartment model since from a mathematical point of view the metabolite can be considered to be the peripheral space. This is clarified if we write down the equations for the system (where index p refers to parent drug):

$$M'(t) = a(t) + k_{mp}M_m(t) - (k_{pm} + k_p)M(t) \qquad (5.16)$$
$$M'_m(t) = a_m(t) + k_{pm}M(t) - (k_{mp} + k_m)M_m(t), \qquad (5.17)$$

Here the rate constants k_{mp} and k_{pm} are conversion rates: e.g., $k_{mp}M_m(t)$ is the amount of metabolite converted to parent drug per time unit. k_p and k_m represent elimination per unit time through other pathways (irreversible metabolic pathways or renal excretion). For the previous discussion on the two-compartment model we only assumed administration into the central compartment, but here we can allow us to administer both parent drug and the metabolite.

Applying $I(.)$ to these equations gives us

$$(k_{pm} + k_p)I(M) - k_{mp}I(M_m) = D,$$
$$-k_{pm}I(M) + (k_{mp} + k_m)I(M_m) = D_m,$$

the solution of which is, if we let $K = (k_{pm} + k_p)(k_{mp} + k_m) - k_{mp}k_{pm}$ denote the determinant of the system,

$$I(M) = \frac{1}{K}((k_{mp} + k_m)D + k_{mp}D_m),$$

$$I(M_m) = \frac{1}{K}((k_{pm} + k_p)D_m + k_{pm}D).$$

If we give only the parent drug $(D_m = 0)$, we get that

$$I(C) = (k_{mp} + k_m)D/KV,$$

whereas if we give only the metabolite instead $(D = 0)$ we get

$$I(C) = k_{mp}D_m/KV.$$

Here V is the volume of distribution for the parent drug. So these integrals differ, if $k_m \neq 0$. This reflects the fact that when given as metabolite some amount of drug is eliminated before it is converted to the parent drug. Also the MRT differs, depending on whether we give a bolus dose of the parent drug or the metabolite, which can be derived in the same way.

5.3   Three-compartment models

Sometimes two compartments do not suffice to describe the distributional behavior of a drug. By adding one, we get a three-compartment model. The exchange of drug between these three compartments can, in analogy with the two-compartment case, be described by rate constants in the following system of differential equations:

$$M_c'(t) = k_{21}M_2(t) + k_{31}M_3(t) - (k_{12} + k_{13})M_c(t) - k_{10}M_c(t),$$
$$M_2'(t) = k_{12}M_c(t) + k_{32}M_3(t) - (k_{21} + k_{23})M_2(t) - k_{20}M_2(t),$$
$$M_3'(t) = k_{13}M_c(t) + k_{23}M_2(t) - (k_{31} + k_{32})M_3(t) - k_{30}M_3(t),$$

with start condition

$$M_c(0) = D, \quad M_2(0) = M_3(0) = 0.$$

If we solve this system, we find a concentration curve in the central compartment that is described by tri-exponential function

$$C(t) = A_1 e^{-\lambda_1 t} + A_2 e^{-\lambda_2 t} + A_3 e^{-\lambda_3 t},$$

where we can assume that $\lambda_1 > \lambda_2 > \lambda_3 = \lambda_{el}$. However, we can not reconstruct the system (determine the rate constants) from $C(t)$, because the model has 6 parameters, of which one is given by the restriction $A_1 + A_2 + A_3 = D/V_c$. Thus, there only remain 5 parameters to determine the 9 rate constants k_{ab} in the system. The only way this can be done is by eliminating 4 parameters by design. Like in the two-compartment case, we can specify where elimination takes place, which eliminates 2 parameters. But there are still two parameters in excess.

We will illustrate this identification problem by looking at two examples.

Example 5.2

When 3 mg of a certain drug was given as a bolus injection, a plasma concentration (μg/L) curve was obtained which was well approximated by the function

$$C(t) = 64e^{-2.35t} + 6e^{-0.19t} + 30e^{-0.69t}.$$

We see that $V_c = 3000/100 = 30$ liters, which is so large that it probably includes both liver and kidneys and we therefore assume that the drug is eliminated from the central compartment. In other words, we assume that

$$k_{20} = k_{30} = 0.$$

There remain seven parameters, so we need to determine two more constants by design. If we restrict ourselves to compartment model with bidirectional flows[1] between compartments we get two different compartmental models, because of the symmetry of the two peripheral compartments (we cannot see them separately, since we only see what happens in the central compartment):

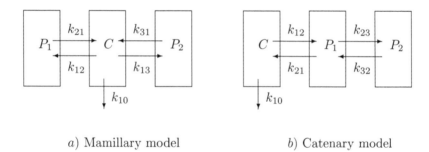

a) Mamillary model   b) Catenary model

FIGURE 5.3: Possible three-compartment models with central elimination

Mamillary model: For this model we assume that the two peripheral compartments communicate only with the central compartment, and not directly with each other. That means that we assume that $k_{32} = k_{23} = 0$.

---

[1]Thereby excluding a case where a drug molecule that goes from the central compartment into the first peripheral compartment must pass also the second peripheral compartment before returning to the central

Catenary model: This model assumes the two peripheral spaces to lie in series, so that the central compartment only communicates with the first peripheral compartment, and that the second peripheral compartment only communicates with the first, but not the central compartment. This means that we assume that $k_{31} = k_{13} = 0$.

For each of these models we now can determine the remaining rate constants, though we do not give the details here. The result is shown in the table below.

Model	k_{10}	k_{12}	k_{13}	k_{21}	k_{23}	k_{31}	k_{32}
Catenary:	0.9776	0.7448	.	0.9569	0.2213	.	0.3293
Mamillary:	0.9776	0.5228	0.2220	1.2569	.	0.2507	.

We can note that some information is the same. For example, the clearance is $CL_c = V_c k_{10} = 29.3$ L/h in both cases, and the distributional clearance $CL_d = V_c(k_{12} + k_{13}) = 22.3$ is also the same for both models.

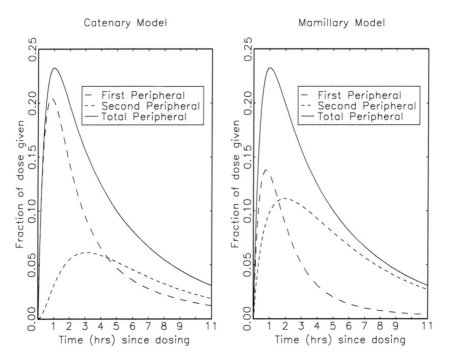

FIGURE 5.4: The distribution between the two peripheral spaces for the two types of three-compartment models with central elimination

The way in which these two models differ is illustrated in Figure 5.4, which shows the total fraction of dose given that is found in the total peripheral space, which is the same for the two models, and how the two models distribute this differently between the two compartments making up the peripheral space.

For future reference, we leave it to the reader to verify that the volume in steady state is estimated to 69.0 liters and that the mean residence time is estimated to 2.35 hours (both of these are estimated from the tri-exponential function defining the plasma concentration only). □

How trustworthy are partitions of drug in the peripheral space into subspaces, like in Figure 5.4? We can illustrate that by estimating a three compartment model to our perfusion-limited physiological model of Section 4.4.2 as given by the concentrations shown in Figure 4.4. This entails a parametric approximation as a mamillary three-compartment model to data we know is not such by design. However, as we see in the left subplot of Figure 5.5, had we had fewer data-points and some noise in the concentration measurements, we would probably think the tri-exponential provides an excellent fit.

To the right in Figure 5.5 we see how the dose given is divided between compartments at different time points. This should be compared with Figure 4.5. From the latter we would expect to pick up one curve containing everything except muscles and adipose tissue as the central compartment, and the two named as the two peripheral compartments. In fact, from the tri-exponential function we get the estimate 17 liters for the volume of the central compartment, which supports this, and the two graphs are in reasonable agreement. In fact, the slowest phase is estimated to have a rate constant of 0.0029, which should be compared to the adipose tissue rate 0.0051 in Example 4.4, and the middle phase has a rate constant estimated to 0.017, which is the same as the rate constant for muscle in Example 4.4.

There are also other possible kinds of non-uniqueness. The next example shows that it is possible that there is more than one set of parameters fitting a given plasma concentration curve for a given model.

Example 5.3

When 0.5 mg of another drug was given as a bolus dose, the following plasma concentration (μg/L) was found:

$$56.313e^{-2.161t} + 22.932e^{-0.578t} + 2.056e^{-0.075t}$$

We see that the central compartment only is about 6.1 liters, which is so small that we assume that the drug is eliminated not from the central compartment, but from one of the peripheral ones.

We assume a *mamillary* model, and that elimination occurs from the first peripheral space. But even then the model is not unique in this case. The system that defines the relation between the tri-exponential function and the

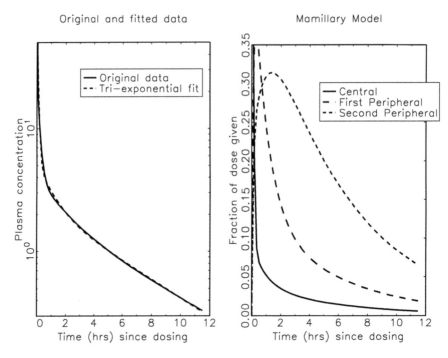

FIGURE 5.5: Fit of an estimated mamillary three-compartment model to the physiological perfusion-limited model. To the right is shown the fraction of the given dose of drug in the different compartments at different time points.

description as a compartmental model with rate constants is non-linear, and in this case it turns out there are two solutions to this:

	k_{21}	k_{12}	k_{31}	k_{13}	k_{20}
Model 1	0.38912	1.38709	0.10231	0.27449	0.66060
Model 2	0.02448	1.14750	1.04977	0.51410	0.07776

We can note from the table that there is one parameter that stays the same for the two models:

$$Cl_d = V_c(k_{12} + k_{13}) = \left\{ \begin{array}{l} 6.1(1.3871 + 0.2745) \\ 6.1(1.1475 + 0.5141) \end{array} \right\} = 10.2 \text{ L/h.}$$

We see that the elimination rate k_{20} of the first model is much larger than that of the second one. So we expect that there will be more drug in the peripheral space in the second model. This is shown in Figure 5.6, which shows the total fraction of drug in the peripheral space, and how this is distributed between the two compartments.   ☐

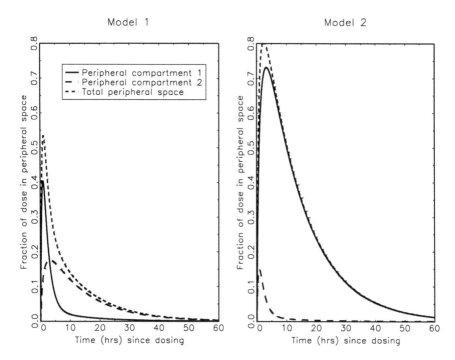

FIGURE 5.6: The peripheral distribution for a plasma concentration that can be expressed as two different mamillary three-compartment models

These two examples show that with three compartments, assumptions must be made that typically are not verifiable. It is also a question of whether these assumptions really produce any useful information – do the rate constants really mean anything to us? Perhaps the only conclusions we should draw are conclusions that can uniquely be derived from the information at hand, which may only be the dose given and the plasma concentration data.

We will now show that we can describe the three-compartment model in the same way as we described the two-compartment model in Section 5.2.3. First we rewrite the equation for the central compartment as

$$V_c C'(t) = k_{21} M_2(t) + k_{31} M_3(t) - CL_d C(t) - CL_c C(t),$$

and consider the remaining two equations as a 2-by-2-system in

$$x(t) = \begin{pmatrix} M_2(t) \\ M_3(t) \end{pmatrix},$$

namely

$$x'(t) = b_2 C(t) + A x(t), \qquad x(0) = 0,$$

with

$$A = \begin{pmatrix} -k_{21} - k_{23} & k_{32} \\ k_{23} & -k_{31} - k_{32} \end{pmatrix} \quad \text{and} \quad b_2 = V_c \begin{pmatrix} k_{12} \\ k_{13} \end{pmatrix}.$$

We can write the solution of this as

$$x(t) = \int_0^t (e^{-A(t-s)} b_2) C(s) ds.$$

This means that if we define

$$h(t) = k_{21} M_2(t) + k_{31} M_3(t) = b_1 e^{-At} b_2, \qquad b_1 = (k_{21} \ k_{31}),$$

(b_1 is a row vector) we can rewrite our equation for the central compartment as

$$V_c C'(t) = (h * C)(t) - CL_d C(t) - CL_c C(t),$$

which is the same equation for the central space as in Section 5.2.3, except that $h(t)$ is now a biexponential function.

Now consider the amount in the total peripheral space, $M_p(t) = M_2(t) + M_3(t)$. With $e = (1 \ 1)$ we then have that

$$M_p'(t) = CL_d C(t) + eA M_p(t).$$

If we introduce the vector u through the relation $eA = -b_1 - u$ and let $e(t) = u^T e^{-At} b_2$ (where T refers to transpose), we get that

$$M_p'(t) = CL_d C(t) - (h * C)(t) - (e * C)(t).$$

Note that

$$M'(t) = V_c C'(t) + M_p'(t) = -CL_c C(t) - (e * C)(t),$$

from which we deduce that $e(t)$ describes the peripheral elimination and that clearance can be written

$$CL(t) = CL_c + (e * C)(t)/C(t).$$

The function $e(t)$ is also a bi-exponential function and is another linear combination of the exponentials that make up $h(t)$.

We now look at the two examples in this section from the perspective just described. The discussion above shows us how knowledge of rate constants, which is what we have from our examples, leads to knowledge of the functions $h(t)$ and $e(t)$. The detailed computations are not shown.

Example 5.4
To continue Example 5.2, for both the catenary and the mamillary model we find the same function $h(t)$:

$$h(t) = 19.712 e^{-1.257t} + 1.670 e^{-0.251t}. \tag{5.18}$$

This function describes the transport of drug through the peripheral space.

For Example 5.3, which assumed peripheral elimination, we have two sets of rate constants to analyze. For both of them one finds that the function $h(t)$ is given by

$$h(t) = 0.055e^{-1.050t} + 0.003e^{-0.102t}. \tag{5.19}$$

The difference between the two models lies in the peripheral excretion function $e(t)$, which is given by

$$e(t) = 0.094e^{-1.050t}$$

for the first model, and

$$e(t) = 0.009e^{-0.102t}$$

for the second model. We see that the excretion rate is much slower for the second model – it is 10 times higher for the first as compared to the second. Without actually sampling from the peripheral space in question, we cannot tell which is the "true" result. ▯

5.4 A general model for distribution and elimination

5.4.1 The model

We have seen that there are uniqueness problems with compartmental models, so instead of persuing the compartmental modelling approach we now formulate a model which is sufficiently rich for most situations. This approach to modelling will use integro-differential equations of the type that has been discussed for both the two- and three-compartment models. We divide the body into a central compartment of volume V_c in which we can measure the concentration $C(t)$, and a peripheral space, that does not need to be homogenous. We assume a bolus dose D given.

The model consists of the two constants V_c, volume of central compartment, and CL_d, the distributional clearance, a description of the central elimination as a clearance function $CL_c(t)$ and two other functions: a function $h(t)$ which describes the transfer through the peripheral space defined implicitly in the equation

$$V_c C'(t) = (h * C)(t) - CL_d C(t) - CL_c(t)C(t), \tag{5.20}$$

and a function $e(t)$ describing the peripheral elimination through the clearance equation

$$CL(t) = CL_c(t) + (e * C)(t)/C(t). \tag{5.21}$$

These two equations constitute the whole model. If we have only central elimination we have $e = 0$ and therefore only one equation.

There are some assumptions in this. We allow for the possibility of capacity limited central elimination, since we make no restriction on $CL_c(t)$. But the distributional processes, as well as the peripheral elimination, are linear processes.

To understand equations 5.20 and 5.21, an alternative description may be helpful. Let T be the stochastic variable that describes the time it takes for a molecule to pass through the peripheral space, i.e., the time from entry to either elimination or return to the central space. Let $S(t) = P(T > t)$ be the survival distribution function for T. Then the amount $M_p(t)$ in the peripheral space is related to the input rate $a_p(t)$ into the peripheral space by the convolution equation

$$M_p(t) = (S * a_p)(t).$$

Differentiation gives us

$$M'_p(t) = a_p(t) + (S' * a_p)(t),$$

which shows that the rate of change of amount of drug in the peripheral space is the difference of the input rate, $a_p(t)$, and the output rate, $(-S' * a_p)(t)$. If we take the distribution for T to be a mixture of two probability distributions

$$S(t) = p_1 S_1(t) + p_2 S_2(t),$$

where index 1 refers to molecules that re-enter the central space and index 2 to molecules that are eliminated from the peripheral space, we see that the flow from peripheral to central space is given by

$$p_1(S'_1 * a_p)(t) = (p_1 CL_d S'_1 * C)(t).$$

Here we have inserted $a_p(t) = CL_d C(t)$ in the expression to the right. It follows that the functions $h(t)$ and $e(t)$ are given by the expressions

$$h(t) = -p_1 CL_d S'_1(t), \qquad e(t) = -p_2 CL_d S'_2(t). \tag{5.22}$$

These expressions help to explain some of the parameter formulas in the next section.

5.4.2 Basic relations and parameters

We will now to a large extent repeat some calculations made in Section 5.2.2 for the two-compartment model. As for the two-compartment case, it depends on the usage of the $I(.)$ and $E(.)$ operators, now applied to the two basic relations, equation 5.20 and the clearance equation 5.21. Most of the computations can be found in Box 5.3. In analogy with CL_{av} we first define the average central clearance, if elimination from the central compartment should have a time-dependent clearance:

$$CL_{c,av} = \frac{\int_0^\infty CL_c(t)C(t)\,dt}{\int_0^\infty C(t)\,dt}.$$

We also introduce a peripheral clearance by

$$CL_p = \int_0^\infty e(t)dt,$$

since then we get the natural division

$$CL_{av} = CL_{c,av} + CL_p,$$

of the total clearance into its central and peripheral parts. Note that with the notation of equations 5.22 we have that $CL_p = p_2 CL_d$.

Since $e(t)$ is an elimination function, we define the *Mean Elimination Time* from the peripheral space by

$$\text{MET}_p = \frac{\int_0^\infty t e(t)\, dt}{CL_p}.$$

In the notation of equations 5.22 this means that MET_p is the expected value of the $S_2(t)$-distribution. Define the constant

$$\kappa = \frac{\int_0^\infty t CL_c(t)C(t)dt)/\int_0^\infty tC(t)dt + CL_p}{CL_{av}},$$

a constant that is one in the most important case, namely when the central clearance is constant. This includes the case when there is only peripheral clearance. Using this constant we have that, see Box 5.3,

$$\text{MRT} = \kappa \text{MRT}_{app} + \frac{CL_p}{CL_{av}}\text{MET}_p. \tag{5.23}$$

If there is only central elimination this equation carries no information, since then $\kappa = \text{MRT}/\text{MRT}_{app}$.

The computations in Box 5.3 show that

$$CL_d = \int_0^\infty h(t)\, dt + CL_p$$

(the integral is $p_1 CL_d$ in the notation of equations 5.22) and that

$$V_{ss} = V_c + \int_0^\infty th(t)\, dt + CL_p\text{MET}_p. \tag{5.24}$$

It is natural to define the volume (as seen through the central compartment) of the peripheral space as

$$V_{ss,p} = \int_0^\infty th(t)\, dt + CL_p\text{MET}_p,$$

since then we get the equation

$$V_{ss} = V_c + V_{ss,p}.$$

Divide this relation by CL_{av}, and we get an equation that divides the total mean residence time (spent in the body) into the mean residence time spent in the two spaces

$$\text{MRT} = \text{MRT}_c + \text{MRT}_p,$$

where

$$\text{MRT}_c = \int_0^\infty \frac{M_c(t)}{D} dt = \frac{V_c}{CL_{av}},$$

and $\text{MRT}_p = V_{ss,p}/CL_{av}$.

The function $h(t)$ describes transfer through the peripheral space back into the central space. It is therefore convenient to define the *Mean Transit Time* of the peripheral space as

$$\text{MTT}_p = \frac{\int_0^\infty t h(t) dt}{\int_0^\infty h(t) dt},$$

which is the expected value of the $S_1(t)$ distribution in equations 5.22. Then we can use this to get the following expression for the volume of the peripheral space

$$V_{ss,p} = (CL_d - CL_p)\text{MTT}_p + CL_p\text{MET}_p.$$

If we define the fractions

$$I_{circ} = \frac{CL_d - CL_p}{CL_{av}}, \quad I_p = \frac{CL_p}{CL_{av}},$$

we can decompose the mean residence time as

$$\text{MRT} = \text{MRT}_c + I_{circ}\text{MTT}_p + I_p\text{MET}_p.$$

Here the mean residence time is divided additively into time spent in the central compartment, a number of circulations (I_{circ}) each taking the mean transit time, and a final elimination time.

We can define two more parameters:

$$F_p = \frac{\text{MRT}_p}{\text{MRT}} = \frac{V_{ss,p}}{V_{ss}},$$

which measures the fraction of time the drug molecules spend in the peripheral space, and

$$K_p = \frac{\text{MRT}_p}{\text{MRT}_c} = \frac{V_{ss,p}}{V_c},$$

which is a kind of partition coefficient.

Example 5.5

For the data in Example 5.2 we have by assumption that $e(t) = 0$ and the transfer function is given by equation 5.18. It follows that

$$\int_0^\infty h(t)\, dt = 22.3, \quad \int_0^\infty t h(t)\, dt = 39.0.$$

Box 5.3 Derivation of PK parameters in the general model

First note that

$$\int_0^\infty CL(t)C(t)dt = CL_{c,av}I(C) + I(e * C) = (CL_{c,av} + I(e))I(C),$$

and since the left-hand-side is D, we obtain

$$CL_{av} = \frac{D}{I(C)} = CL_{c,av} + I(e) = CL_c + CL_p.$$

Next we compute the integral $\int tCL(t)C(t)dt$:

$$E(CL_cC) + I(e)E(C) + E(e)I(C) = \kappa CL_{av}E(C) + E(e)I(C),$$

with $\kappa = (E(CL_cC)/E(C)+CL_p)/CL_{av}$, and if we divide it by $\int CL(t)C(t)dt$, we obtain

$$\text{MRT} = \frac{\kappa CL_{av}E(C) + E(e)I(C)}{CL_{av}I(C)} = \kappa\frac{E(C)}{I(C)} + \frac{E(e)}{CL_{av}},$$

which gives us equation 5.23. Next, if we apply $I(.)$ to equation 5.20, we get

$$I(h)I(C) - (CL_d + CL_{c,av})I(C) = -D = -CL_{av}I(C)$$

from which we deduce that $CL_d = I(h) + CL_p$. If we instead apply $E(.)$ to it we get

$$-V_cI(C) = I(h)E(C) + E(h)I(C) - CL_dE(C) - E(CL_cC)$$

and if we use that

$$E(CL_cC) = (\kappa CL_{av} - CL_p)E(C)$$

then

$$(V_c + E(h))I(C) = (CL_d - I(h) + \kappa CL_{av} - CL_p)E(C) = \kappa CL_{av}E(C).$$

If we add $E(e)I(C)$ to both sides and divide by $I(C)$, we obtain

$$V_{ss} = CL_{av}\,\text{MRT} = V_c + E(h) + E(e).$$

The distributional clearance CL_d is therefore 22.3 L/h, whereas the volume in steady state of the peripheral space $V_{ss,p}$ is 39.0 liters. Note that our old estimate of V_{ss} at the end of Example 5.2 is precisely the sum of the volume of central space and this. The mean residence time in the central space is estimated (since clearance is estimated in Example 5.2 to 29.3) to $\text{MRT}_c = 30/29.3 = 1.02$ h, and the mean residence time in the peripheral space to $\text{MRT}_p = 39.0/29.3 = 1.33$ h, summing up to our old estimate for MRT in Example 5.2. Moreover the mean transit time of the peripheral space is

$$\text{MTT}_p = 39.0/22.3 = 1.75$$

so we see that the number of circulations is

$$I_{circ} = \frac{\text{MRT}_p}{\text{MTT}_p} = \frac{1.33}{1.75} = 0.76.$$

So on average three out of four molecules enters the peripheral space before being eliminated. Related numbers are that 56.5% of the time is spent in the peripheral space (F_p) and that the partition coefficient between the peripheral and central spaces (K_p) is 1.3. $\quad\square$

Example 5.6
For both models in Example 5.3 we have that the transfer function $h(t)$ is given by Equation 5.19, so

$$\int_0^\infty h(t)\, dt = 4.85, \qquad \int_0^\infty t h(t)\, dt = 19.5.$$

Since we have only peripheral elimination, we have that $CL_p = CL_{av} = 5.4$ L/h, and also that

$$CL_d = I(h) + CL_p = 10.2 \text{ L/h}.$$

The mean transit time of the peripheral space is $\text{MTT}_p = 4.0$ h.

We recall that in Example 5.3 we have two models, one with a slower elimination rate than the other. For Model 1, with the faster elimination rate of the two, we have that MET = 0.95 hours, and for Model 2 we have MET = 9.8 hours. The effect of these differences is shown in the following table, in which CL is computed as $I(e)$ for the two models.

Parameter	NCA	short MET	long MET
CL (L/h)	5.4	5.4	5.4
MRT (h)	4.8	5.7	14.6
V_{ss} (L)	25.7	30.8	78.2

Since the mean residence time in the central compartment is $\text{MRT}_c = 1.15$ h and the circulation number is $I_{circ} = I(h)/CL_{av} = 0.90$, we see that MRT is obtained by adding MET to $\text{MRT}_{app} = \text{MRT}_c + I_{circ}\text{MTT}_p = 1.15 + 0.90 \cdot 4.0 = 4.8$ h. Similarly we obtain the V_{ss} from the NCA analysis from $V_c + E(h)$ to which we should add MET_p to get the true V_{ss}.

5.4.3 Revisiting the two-compartment model

In this section we will re-derive the formulae of Section 5.2 and see what extra information the discussion in the previous section provides us with.

Referring to Section 5.2, we see that we can describe a two-compartment model as equation 5.20 and the clearance equation 5.21 with

$$CL_c(t) = V_c k_{ce}, \quad h(t) = V_c k_{cp} k_{pc} e^{-(k_{pc}+k_{pe})t}, \quad e(t) = V_c k_{cp} k_{pe} e^{-(k_{pc}+k_{pe})t}.$$

From this we can compute the building blocks:

$$\int_0^\infty h(t)dt = V_c \frac{k_{cp} k_{pc}}{k_{pc} + k_{pe}}, \quad \int_0^\infty th(t)dt = V_c \frac{k_{cp} k_{pc}}{(k_{pc} + k_{pe})^2},$$

and the corresponding integrals for $e(t)$ are computed using the observation $e(t) = k_{pc}h(t)/k_{pe}$. Immediate consequences of this are that

$$CL_p = V_c \frac{k_{cp} k_{pe}}{k_{pc} + k_{pe}}, \quad \text{MET}_p = \frac{1}{k_{pc} + k_{pe}}$$

from which we first re-derive that

$$CL_{av} = V_c(k_{ce} + \frac{k_{cp} k_{pe}}{k_{pc} + k_{pe}}).$$

Next, a short computation shows that $CL_d = V_c k_{cp}$ and

$$V_{ss} = V_c(1 + \frac{k_{cp}}{k_{pc} + k_{pe}}).$$

These are our old formulae. We also have the mean transit time through the peripheral space as

$$\text{MTT}_p = \frac{1}{k_{pc} + k_{pe}}$$

and the two circulation indices

$$I_{circ} = \frac{k_{cp} k_{pc}}{k_{ce}(k_{pc} + k_{pe}) + k_{cp} k_{pe}}, \quad I_p = \frac{k_{cp} k_{pe}}{k_{ce}(k_{pc} + k_{pe}) + k_{cp} k_{pe}},$$

and if we plug this into the formula for MRT_p we get, noting that MTT_p and MET_p are the same,

$$\text{MRT}_p = \frac{k_{cp}}{k_{ce}(k_{pc} + k_{pe}) + k_{cp} k_{pe}}.$$

We also have that

$$\text{MRT}_c = \frac{k_{pc} + k_{pe}}{k_{ce}(k_{pc} + k_{pe}) + k_{cp}k_{pe}}$$

and adding them together we retrieve our old formula for MRT.

Example 5.7

We now apply this to the data in Example 2.1. The MTT_p is 1.53 hours and the MRT_c 2.18 hours both when we have central and peripheral elimination, since the sum $k_{pc} + k_{pe}$ is the same in both cases. However the peripheral MRT is larger when we have peripheral elimination: it is 2.39 hours with central and 3.92 hours with peripheral elimination. This is easy to understand: the MET_p is the same as MTT_p, 1.53 hours, and has to be added to MRT_p. But because of this, the fraction of time spent peripherally is larger with peripheral elimination than with central elimination: 0.64 versus 0.52. Finally, the circulation index I_{circ} is 1.57 both for central and peripheral elimination, so that a drug molecule on average passes through the peripheral space 1.57 times before it is eliminated (not counting the final pass in case of peripheral elimination). □

5.4.4 Computing the transfer function

So far we have only investigated for previously defined compartmental models what the general model provides us with. But it can also be used as a part of a non-compartmental approach, provided we can estimate the transfer and peripheral elimination functions from data. In general, as already seen in the two-compartment model, it is not possible to get detailed information about $e(t)$, instead we in general hope for (i.e., assume) central elimination. In this section we will derive formulae which allow us to estimate the transfer function $h(t)$, or, as it turns out, its (negative) primitive function

$$H(t) = \int_t^\infty h(s)ds. \tag{5.25}$$

Using the notations in equation 5.22 we have that $H(t) = CL_d p_1 S_1(t)$.

If we integrate equation 5.20 from t to ∞ we get

$$-V_c C(t) = \int_t^\infty (h * C)(s)ds - CL_d \int_t^\infty C(s)ds - \int_t^\infty CL_c(s)C(s)ds.$$

Using formula 1.7 this can be rewritten as

$$(H * C)(t) + (I(h) - CL_d)\int_t^\infty C(s)ds = \int_t^\infty CL_c(s)C(s)ds - V_c C(t),$$

which in turn can be rearranged to

$$(H * C)(t) = \int_t^\infty (CL_c(s) + CL_p)C(s)ds - V_c C(t). \tag{5.26}$$

With known integrand on the right hand side, we can obtain $H(t)$ by de-convolution from this. In some cases we can do this analytically, as will be discussed below, but in general we may need to do it numerically, using the methods of Section 3.4.

When we describe our plasma concentrations for a bolus dose as a polyexpo-nential function, also the function $H(t)$ is a polyexponential function, with one exponential term less than $C(t)$. We can derive an explicit formula for $H(t)$ in the case when the central clearance is constant. First we rewrite formula 5.26 as

$$(H * C)(t) = CL \int_t^\infty C(s)ds - V_c C(t). \tag{5.27}$$

How to derive a formula for $H(t)$ from this is shown in Box 5.4.

Example 5.8
Let us see how the content of Box 5.4 agrees with what we know about the two-compartment model. This is the case $N = 2$, so the equation for $H(t) = he^{-\gamma t}$ consists of the three equations

$$\frac{A_1}{\gamma - \lambda_1} + \frac{A_2}{\gamma - \lambda_2} = 0, \quad \frac{h}{\gamma - \lambda_i} = \frac{CL_{av}}{\lambda_i} - V_c, i = 1, 2.$$

The first is a linear equation in γ, giving

$$\gamma = \frac{A_1\lambda_2 + A_2\lambda_1}{A_1 + A_2} = \frac{\lambda_1\lambda_2 V_c}{CL_{av}}.$$

Then we can determine h from

$$h = (\frac{CL_{av}}{\lambda_1} - V_c)(\gamma - \lambda_1) = \frac{1}{CL_{av}}(CL_{av} - \lambda_1 V_c)(\lambda_2 V_c - CL_{av}).$$

Plugging in expression 5.7 for CL_{av} and simplifying shows that

$$h = V_c \frac{k_{cp}k_{pc}}{k_{pc} + k_{pe}}, \quad \gamma = k_{pc} + k_{pe},$$

which agrees with what we found in Section 5.2.1. ⬚

Example 5.9
Consider again Example 5.2. In this example we assumed central elimination and constant clearance, so equation 5.27 applies. Note that we already have an analytic expression for $H(t)$ by integrating equation 5.18. We know that $CL = 29.3$ and $V_c = 30$ so we can also use the explicit representation of the plasma concentration as a tri-exponential function and use these parameters to give an analytic expression for the right hand side of equation 5.27 and

---

Box 5.4 Deriving the transfer function for plasma concentrations described by poly-exponentials

---

If $C(t)$ is a polyexponential, the function $H(t)$ in formula 5.25 is also polyexponential, but with one term less, as we will now see. Assume

$$C(t) = \sum_{i=1}^{N} A_i e^{-\lambda_i t}, \quad H(t) = \sum_{j=1}^{N-1} h_j e^{-\gamma_j t}.$$

Then

$$(H * C)(t) = \sum_{i,j} A_i h_j e^{-\gamma_j t} \int_0^t e^{(\gamma_j - \lambda_i)s} ds = \sum_{i,j} \frac{A_i h_j}{\gamma_j - \lambda_i} (e^{-\lambda_i t} - e^{-\gamma_j t}),$$

$$CL_{av} \int_t^\infty C(s) ds - V_c C(t) = \sum_{i=1}^{N} A_i (\frac{CL_{av}}{\lambda_i} - V_c) e^{-\lambda_i t}.$$

We can therefore re-write the equation as

$$\sum_{i=1}^{N} (\sum_{j=1}^{N-1} \frac{A_i h_j}{\gamma_j - \lambda_i}) e^{-\lambda_i t} - \sum_{j=1}^{N-1} h_j \sum_{i=1}^{N} (\frac{A_i}{\gamma_j - \lambda_i}) e^{-\gamma_j t} = \sum_{i=1}^{N} A_i (\frac{CL_{av}}{\lambda_i} - V_c) e^{-\lambda_i t}.$$

By identification, it follows that the coefficients $\gamma_i, i = 1, \ldots, N-1$ are determined from the equations

$$\sum_{i=1}^{N} \frac{A_i}{\gamma_j - \lambda_i} = 0, j = 1, \ldots, N-1.$$

Then the coefficients h_j are determined through the relation

$$\sum_{j=1}^{N-1} \frac{h_j}{\gamma_j - \lambda_i} = \frac{CL_{av}}{\lambda_i} - V_c, i = 1, \ldots, N.$$

---

then numerically solve equation 5.27 for $H(t)$. We do that by computing the right hand side at the time points $0.25, 0.5, 1$ and then every hour up to 12. Based on this data we now make a numerical deconvolution, using the trapeze method, which provides us with estimates of $H(t)$. The result is shown in Figure 5.7 which also shows the analytical function for comparison.

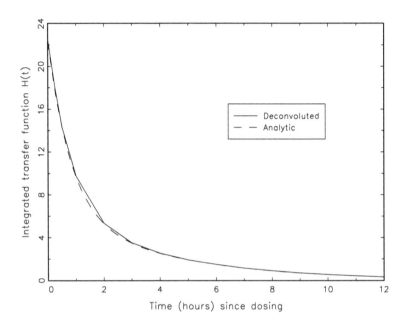

FIGURE 5.7: True and numerically estimated integrated transfer function for three-compartment model

To estimate $I(h)$ is simple. It is given by $H(0) = 22.4$, and by numerical integration of $H(t)$ (again using the trapeze formula) we can estimate $E(h) = I(H) = 38.7$. These numbers are close, but of course not identical, to the numbers we obtained by analytical methods earlier. In fact, in estimating $I(H)$ we used the trapeze formula over the observational time interval only, not including the extrapolation using a monoexponential function which is needed for the full integral to be computed. ▯

An alternative formulation of Equation 5.26 is

$$((H + E) * C)(t) = \int_t^\infty CL(s)C(s)ds - V_cC(t),$$

which can be derived by the corresponding integration of the clearance equation. The right hand side of this equation is the amount of drug still to be eliminated, minus what is in the central space. In other words:

$$M_p(t) = ((H + E) * C)(t).$$

This allows us an independent justification for formula 5.24 for the volume in steady state. If we keep the plasma concentration of drug at a constant level C, the previous formula tells us that the amount of drug peripherally is given by $M_p = I(H + E)C$, so the total amount of drug in the body is $M = V_cC + I(H + E)C$. Since $I(H + E) = E(h) + E(e)$, this shows that

$$V_{ss} = \frac{M}{C} = V_c + E(h) + E(e),$$

which is the same as formula 5.24.

Example 5.10
We now apply this analysis to the venous concentration curve obtained from the perfusion limited physiological model in Example 4.4 in order to see what information we obtain. The distribution parameter estimates are:

CL_d	I_{circ}	$V_{ss,p}$ (L)	MRT$_c$ (h)	MRT$_p$ (h)	MTT$_p$ (min)	F_p	K_p
3784	5	170	0.15	3.8	45	96	25

We see that the distributional clearance (mL/min) is five times larger than the elimination clearance (the estimated value of I_{circ}) and that most time is spent in the peripheral space. We also see that the volume of the peripheral space is correctly estimated, since the central space is about 7 L. What may be surprising is the mean transit time of the peripheral space, which is larger than the circulation time obtained in Example 4.6. At first sight this may appear contradictory and may be attributed to problems with estimating the function $H(t)$. The following discussion shows that this is not the case.

We saw in Section 4.4.2 that the NCA analysis, of which the present analysis is an extension, identifies a central space consisting of blood vessels, lungs, and kidneys. Summing up the equations for these four organs, we find that the concentration $C(t)$ in the central space (which is equal to the venous concentration) is given by

$$V_cC'(t) = \sum_{i \in I} Q_iC_i(t) - Q_cC(t),$$

where the kidneys are taken out of the index set I of organs with output on the venous side and therefore Q_c is the cardiac output minus the kidney blood flow, which is 4160 mL/min. Since elimination occurs peripherally, in the liver, this therefore is the true distributional clearance, CL_d.

There is an analytical formula for the mean transit time of the peripheral space for this model:

$$\text{MTT}_p = \frac{\sum_i Q_i \text{MTT}_i - E(Q_{liver}\text{MTT}_{liver} + Q_{GI}\text{MTT}_{GI})}{Q_c - EQ_{liver}}. \tag{5.28}$$

The derivation can be found in Box 5.5. Inserting the parameters from Table 4.1 here we find that $\text{MTT}_p = 48$ minutes.

This may seem surprising at first, since we have seen in Example 4.4 that the total circulation time is less than this, only 37 minutes. However, the two models should not be confused. Circulation in the original model involved passing veins-lungs-arteries, which took on average 1.2 minutes to pass, and then one of the visceral organs. In the present model, the kidneys are part of the central space. In the original model, 22% of the visceral flow passed the kidneys in which they had a transit time of only 0.30 minutes. It follows that we should have, approximately since we ignore elimination,

$$1.2 + 0.22 \cdot 0.30 + 0.78\text{MTT}_p = 37,$$

or $\text{MTT}_p = 46$ minutes. □

5.5 Example: Distribution analysis of budesonide and fluticasone

We now apply the analysis of the distribution processes described in the previous section to the data of the two steroids budesonide and fluticasone discussed in example 3.6. Recall that the size of the volume of the central compartment leads us to believe that we have central elimination, in which case we know that all our parameters are derived from the two integrals, with $H(t)$ defined in formula 5.25,

$$\int_0^\infty h(t)\,dt = H(0), \qquad \int_0^\infty th(t)\,dt = \int_0^\infty H(t)\,dt.$$

We also know that the second of these can be calculated as

$$\int_0^\infty th(t)\,dt = V_{ss,p} = V_{ss} - V_c,$$

where we have the two volume parameters on the right hand side already. However, the first integral cannot be calculated in a similar way. We assume that clearance is constant, so that equation 5.27 applies.

We first estimate the function $H(t)$ by numerical deconvolution of equation 5.27. In this equation $C(t)$ refers to plasma concentrations after a bolus

---

Box 5.5 Derivation of the mean transit time of the peripheral space for a physiological model

---

The peripheral space is made up of five spaces lying in parallel, four of which are compartments. The remaining one is the intestine-liver system. For each organ except the liver, but including the intestines, we have that $C_i = H_i * C$, where $H_i(t) = k_i e^{-k_i t}$ and k_i is the tissue rate constant. For the liver we can rewrite the equation as

$$V_i K_{p,i} C_i'(t) = Q_i((H_{in} * C)(t) - C_i(t)/(1 - E))$$

where

$$H_{in}(t) = \frac{Q_{ha}}{Q_i} \delta_0 + \frac{Q_{pv}}{Q_i} H_{GI}(t).$$

Here δ_0 is the Dirac measure, i.e., a point mass in the origin and we have that

$$I(H_{in}) = \frac{Q_{ha}}{Q_i} + \frac{Q_{pv}}{Q_i} I(H_{GI}) = 1, \quad E(H_{in}) = \frac{Q_{pv}}{Q_i} E(H_{GI}) = \frac{V_{GI} K_{p,GI}}{Q_i}.$$

It follows that for the liver we have

$$C_i = (H_i * H_{in}) * C \text{ where } H_i(t) = k_i e^{-k_i t/(1-E)}.$$

From this we deduce that

$$\sum_{i \in I} Q_i C_i(t) = (h * C)(t)$$

where, with $I' = \{\text{brain, muscles, adipose tissue, skin}\}$,

$$h(t) = Q_{liver}(H_{liver} * H_{in})(t) + \sum_{i \in I'} Q_i H_i(t).$$

This is therefore the transfer function of the peripheral space. Note that

$$I(h) = \sum_{i \in I'} Q_i + Q_{liver}(1 - E) = Q_c - E Q_{liver},$$

and that

$$E(h) = Q_{liver}((1 - E) E(H_{in}) + E(H_{liver})) + \sum_{i \in I'} Q_i E(H_i),$$

from which we can deduce the analytic expression in formula 5.28 for the mean transit time of the peripheral space.

---

dose and not after a 10 minute infusion which is how our data were obtained. The connection between the concentration after a unit bolus dose, $G(t)$, and the concentration after an infusion of dose D for an infusion time τ was given in formula 2.14. For a short infusion time that gives us the approximation

$$G(t_i - \tau/2) \approx (G_*(t_i) - G_*(t_i - \tau))/\tau = C(t_i)/D.$$

Using this we can estimate the right hand side of equation 5.27 numerically and solve the convolution equation. The functions $H(t)$ so obtained are displayed in Figure 5.8.

Based on $H(0)$ (and the integral of $H(t)$) we compute the distribution parameters discussed in the previous section. For each of these and each steroid, the geometric means, with confidence intervals, together with their ratios are summarized in Table 5.1.

What we see in Table 5.1 is first that the distributional clearance is twice as large for budesonide as for fluticasone. However, from Figure 5.8 we also see that the time spent in the peripheral space is much shorter. In fact, we see that MTT_p is four times larger for fluticasone than for budesonide. But the peripheral mean residence time is only about twice as large for fluticasone as for budesonide.

This is as much as we can say from the available data. If we want to say more, we must make additional assumptions. From the various graphs showing the intravenous data, including Figure 5.8, we see that data should be fairly accurately described by a tri-exponential function. If we do that, we can build compartmental models that may provide some further information which may be of interest. We will make such an exploration here in order to illustrate how the content of this chapter fits together.

We will do that based on the (geometric) mean value curves. We have seen that these do represent a typical individual curve in this particular case. Fitting a tri-exponential function with a 10 minute infusion to such mean data provides an almost perfect fit as is shown in Figure 5.9.

The half-lives for each of the three phases are shown in the following table

	Half-life for phase		
Steroid	first (min)	second (h)	third (h)
Budesonide	2.29	1.28	4.51
Fluticasone	2.34	1.17	11.65

The first two phases appear very similar for the two steroids, but the numerical differences are visible in Figure 5.9. The main difference, however, lies in the last phase, as we already knew from an earlier analysis. In order to translate this into compartmental models we need to decide on a choice of model.

For fluticasone, which is a highly lipophilic substance, it is reasonable to assume that cell membranes pose very little barrier to diffusion, and that what we see in terms of phases in the tri-exponential approximation is the result of

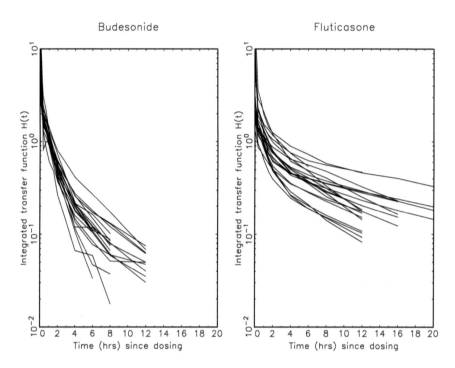

FIGURE 5.8: The integrated transfer functions $H(t)$ through the peripheral space

Table 5.1: Disposition parameters for the two steroids

Parameter	Budesonide		Fluticasone		Mean Ratio	
	mean	95% C.I.	mean	95% C.I.	ratio	95% C.I.
CL_d (mL/min)	6513	(4709, 9009)	3655	(2622, 5094)	0.561	(0.358, 0.88)
$V_{ss,p}$ (L)	293	(270, 318)	677	(565, 812)	2.31	(1.91, 2.8)
MRT_c (h)	0.336	(0.274, 0.413)	0.224	(0.178, 0.282)	0.665	(0.493, 0.897)
MRT_p (h)	3.49	(3.14, 3.88)	8.24	(6.71, 10.1)	2.36	(1.89, 2.95)
MTT_p (h)	0.749	(0.531, 1.06)	3.09	(2.24, 4.26)	4.12	(2.61, 6.5)
F_p (%)	90.3	(88, 92.6)	97	(96.3, 97.7)	1.07	(1.05, 1.1)
K_p	10.4	(8.3, 13)	36.9	(29.2, 46.5)	3.55	(2.6, 4.85)

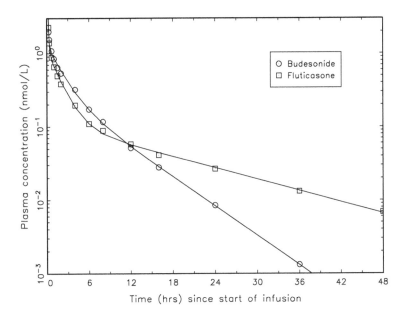

FIGURE 5.9: Tri-exponential approximation of mean infusion data

perfusion limitations. Based on our previous discussion of such models, this would justify a mamillary model for this drug.

Budesonide, on the other hand, is a soluble, less lipophilic, substance. Crossing membranes may therefore be more of a problem. We know that it passes cell membranes, because the steroid receptor is an intracellular protein, not one on the cell membrane. Since the plasma concentration declines rapidly after administration we may assume that the vascular walls are passed easily so that the first phase essentially means distribution in the interstitial space. The second phase would then be intracellular distribution. But what, then, is the third phase? Evidence emerged during the 1990's that there is a reversible intracellular esterification of budesonide. These fatty acid conjugates of budesonide could act as inactive intracellular stores of the steroid and they could be considered a third compartment (which then is not a space, but a biochemical transformation). This would justify a catenary model for budesonide.

After having estimated these three-compartment models from the tri-exponentials we can draw the graphs in Figure 5.10. It shows the fraction of drug administered that is found within the different compartments, plus a solid curve showing the fraction of drug found anywhere in the body. The last curve is independent of choice of model. In fact, it can be obtained within

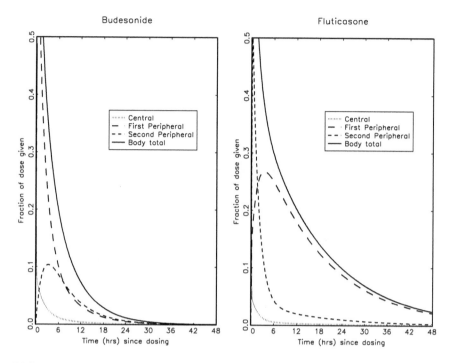

FIGURE 5.10: Fraction of drug in body and the three suggested compartments

the non-compartmental approach from the formula

$$M(t) = CL \int_t^\infty C(t)\,dt, \quad t > 10 \text{ min.}$$

We see that the lipophilic fluticasone is retained in the body substantially longer than budesonide, despite considerably lower plasma concentrations. This explains why there is a much more pronounced accumulation for fluticasone than for budesonide on multiple dosing. We also see that for fluticasone there is one compartment into which drug is drawn and which has a small tissue rate constant. This rate constant therefore determines the terminal elimination rate. It is tempting to think that this at least contains adipose tissue.

For budesonide on the other hand we note the curve describing the second peripheral compartment, which according to our modelling should be the ester forms of budesonide. From the rate constants we find that the rate of ester formation is 0.12 per hour, whereas the reverse operation, splitting steroid and ester, proceeds with a rate of 0.26 per hour. It is this last step which ultimately determines the observed terminal elimination rate in plasma.

But all this is speculation. The author asks the reader to consider this discussion a description of how modelling can be done, not as an accurate description of the true nature of the steroids analyzed.

One final point to make is the following. In the description above we fitted our tri-exponential model to mean data (on the logarithmic scale). This was done for convenience only, and it means that we described the mean value curve, not the mean parameter curve, which is a typical subject curve. An analysis of the mean parameter curve instead can be made in complete analogy with what was done above, except that we start by fitting the same model function to data using the appropriate NonLinear Mixed Effects Model estimation method. In this case the difference is not great [2], and the overall description is about the same.

5.6 Chapter epilogue: The distribution model and the recirculation model

We can now tie the recirculation model first discussed in Section 2.6 to the distribution model discussed in this chapter, based on equation 5.20. This has already been done to some extent when we have discussed pharmacokinetic analysis of the perfusion limited physiological model. One assumption of the recirculation model is that we do not have any non-linearities, so in equation 5.20 we should have a constant central clearance. Write temporarily $K = (CL_d + CL_c)/V_c$ and $h_.(t) = h(t)/V_c$. Equation 5.20 then takes the form

$$C'(t) = (h_. * C)(t) - KC(t).$$

Note that we assume a bolus dose, so that $C(0) = D/V_c$. We can rewrite this equation as a convolution equation

$$C(t) = C(0)e^{-Kt} + (e^{-Kt} * h_. * C)(t).$$

If we compare this expression with that of equation 2.20, we see that the one-pass circulation function is given by

$$H(t) = \int_0^t e^{-K(t-s)} h(s) \, ds/V_c,$$

and that $a(t) = C(0)e^{-Kt}$.

Focussing on the one-pass circulation function we find that

$$I(H) = \frac{I(h)}{V_c K} = \frac{CL_d - CL_p}{CL_d + CL_c}$$

from which we deduce that the body extraction ratio is given by

$$E = \frac{CL}{CL_d + CL_c}.$$

A short computation shows that the circulation time is given by

$$t_{circ} = \frac{E(H)}{I(H)} = \text{MTT}_p + \frac{1}{K},$$

which says that it is the sum of the mean time spent in the peripheral space and in the central space.

When we insert here numbers obtained in the analysis made in Example 5.10, we find a much larger extraction ratio and larger circulation time compared to what we found in the direct analysis done at the end of Example 4.4. The difference between the two approaches is that in the recirculation analysis made in Example 4.4 we used the true value for $C(0)$, whereas in the NCA analysis that preceded it, and was continued in Example 5.10, we extrapolated a value for this backward from 1 and 2 minute data. But we have seen that this leads to different views on the size of the central compartment - the true size is the volume of the veins whereas extrapolation defines a space containing both that and the arteries, plus both lungs and kidneys. This is the difference between the abstract bolus dose and what we actually can measure. But the recirculation model, in order to provide correct data, needs an accurate start concentration. In real life we cannot obtain such accuracy. If we redo the NCA analysis of the physiological model, including the extension in Example 5.10, with the true start concentration, we do get correct numbers.

Chapter 6

PK/PD modelling

6.1 Therapeutic response

Previous chapters have discussed how the body handles a drug we take as a treatment, but they also apply to things like alcohol and caffeine that we take for reasons we seldom consider therapeutic. The reason we take the drug is that we want some kind of therapeutic response to it, a response that often is the result of drug-receptor interaction, either on or within some (or all) cell types. It is unbound drug that can bind to receptors and the likelihood of this to happen increases with dose given, since this should increase the number of free molecules per volume unit in the vicinity of the receptors, i.e., the local concentration of drug at what may be called the *effect site*.

The drug concentration at the effect site should bear some relation to the plasma concentration which we can measure. The description of the time evolution of effect after dosing of a drug is what pharmacodynamics (abbreviated PD) is about. Modelling the relationship between plasma concentrations and effect is called PK/PD modelling. Using that information, we can find the appropriate dosage regimen of the drug. The ultimate objective of this is to build a function that transforms a dosage regimen to a therapeutic response profile.

In reality there may be too many factors which contribute to the response, so we may have to be content with a rather crude model. That, on the other hand, may be sufficient for the purpose we have, which is to find the appropriate dosage regimen. In this chapter we will only address pharmacodynamic modelling from an empirical point of view when more detailed knowledge of the processes that lead from the plasma concentrations to the response is not sufficient for detailed modelling.

Information gathering for this type of modelling typically passes three stages. First we make *in vitro* experiments, which include studying drug-enzyme kinetics alone or in isolated tissue or organ. This is a much simpler situation than that of a living being, where complex interrelationships may play a complicating part. The effects of such complications are studied in step two, which consists of animal experiments, before we make the last series of studies, the human experiments. In animals we can, among other things, study doses which, in relation to body weight, we can never study in humans, allowing us to get toxicity information. There are two kinds of toxicities involved: those that are predicted from the pharmacological effect of the drug, and those that appear unexpectedly, because the structure of the molecule happens to lead to effects which were not part of the target profile, or it was metabolized to something that had such effects.

Almost all drugs have unwanted side-effects at enough high doses, and all drugs need a minimum dose to give any noticeable response. Thus, all drugs have some kind of *therapeutic window* of doses, and for many drugs this is measured as therapeutic plasma concentrations instead, as was briefly discussed in Section 2.4.

There are two main, but opposite, ways in which a drug works.

- It can be a man-made analogue to a naturally occurring (endogenous) molecule in the body which, when binding to a particular receptor, has an effect similar to the latter. Such drugs are called *agonists*.

- It can be designed to bind to a particular receptor but have no effect, thereby preventing an endogenous molecule from binding and having an effect. Such drugs are called *antagonists*. It is a *competitive antagonist* if it binds reversibly to the receptor.

In the following sections we will study some aspects of the mathematical analysis of agonists and antagonists. First we will do that in situations that are more like *in vitro* experiments, in which we control the drug concentrations and hold them fixed at different levels. After that we will look into how we can approach the problem of linking effect to varying drug concentrations.

6.2   Modelling a simple agonist

Many drugs are designed as simple agonists to existing endogenous substances. This means that there are receptors on or within some cells, ready to bind to them, and with consequences in those cells which are the same as the endogenous substance has. They are man-made analogues of what nature has invented. The simplest model for such a drug D is that it binds reversibly to the receptor sites R and that the complex DR exerts some effect. According to the *receptor occupancy hypothesis*, the size of the effect is some function, the *intrinsic activity*, of the number of bound complexes:

$$E = f([DR])$$

where E is the effect measured on some scale and $f(u)$ a function such that $f(0) = 0$. The dynamics behind receptor binding is the same as behind protein binding (receptors are proteins - the only difference is that these proteins are within the cells or on their membranes):

$$D + R \underset{k_{-1}}{\overset{k_1}{\rightleftharpoons}} DR,$$

which, using the law of mass action, leads to the differential equation

$$[DR]' = k_1[R][D] - k_{-1}[DR], \quad [R] + [DR] = R_0,$$

where R_0 is the concentration of all receptor sites. We can rewrite this as

$$[DR]' = k_1 R_0[D] - (k_{-1} + k_1[D])[DR], \tag{6.1}$$

and if we hold $C = [D]$ constant, this can be solved to

$$[DR](t) = \frac{k_1 R_0 C}{k_{-1} + k_1 C}(1 - \exp(-(k_{-1} + k_1 C)t)).$$

At equilibrium we find

$$[DR] = \frac{R_0 C}{K_d + C}, \quad K_d = \frac{k_{-1}}{k_1}, \tag{6.2}$$

where the constant K_d is called the *dissociation constant*. In the context of protein binding in Section 4.2.1, we encountered its inverse, the association constant K_a, which measures the affinity of the drug to the receptor.

If we, furthermore, assume that the response we get is proportional (over the range in question) to the number of complexes ($f(u) = ku$ for some k), we end up with the *concentration-effect relationship*

$$E(C) = \frac{E_{max} C}{EC_{50} + C}, \quad EC_{50} = K_d. \tag{6.3}$$

The notation EC_{50} indicates that K_d in fact is the concentration that gives half the maximum effect. It measures the *potency* of the drug. When drug potencies are compared, what is compared is the concentrations that produce the same effect, not the magnitudes of effect at the same concentration. The number E_{max} is called the *efficacy* of the drug-receptor complex and gives the maximal effect attainable. In this simple model this occurs when all receptors are bound to drug.

Not all pharmacologically interesting receptors are within the cell membranes. The glucocorticosteroids discussed in Section 3.6, for example, bind to intracellular receptors which interact with so-called transcription factors that help in gene regulation. Thus such drugs need to enter cells to have an effect.

The model described so far is probably too simple in most instances: many receptors reside within the cell membrane and in order to be able to exert

Box 6.1 Outline of the β_2-adrenoreceptor

The β_2-adrenergic receptors are found in the cell membranes of the smooth muscles lining the airways of the lungs. They are the target for, e.g., the hormone adrenaline, and therefore also the target for β_2-agonists, the rescue medication asthmatics use, which are man-made analogues of adrenaline. They are also found in other cell types in the body.

The binding of a β_2-agonist to this receptor causes a structural change in the receptor protein. The β_2-agonist has seven transmembrane domains which are associated with a so-called G protein in the cell membrane. When the receptor is activated, it causes a conformal change in the G protein. A GDP (guanosine 5'-diphosphate) group associated with the G protein then becomes dissociated and is replaced with a GTP (guanosine 5'-triphosphate) group. This in turn causes one of the three sub units (the α unit) to dissociate from the G complex and to freely move in the membrane. This sub-unit can activate the enzyme adenyl cyclase, which catalyzes the conversion of ATP to cAMP (adenosine 5'-triphosphate to cyclic adenosine 3',5'-monophosphate).

The increased cAMP levels in the cell activates another enzyme, protein kinase A, which transfers the terminal phosphate group of an ATP to several target proteins within the cell. One of the effects of this is the active transport of Ca^{2+} ions into intracellular stores. This lowers the intracellular free Ca^{2+} concentrations of the smooth muscles, leading to muscle relaxation. Muscle contraction is initiated by a rise in intracellular free Ca^{2+} concentrations, because the ion activates certain enzymes.

The effect subsides when GTP is hydrolised to GDP and the α-unit reconvenes with the other two units of the G-protein.

some effect within the cell, the drug-receptor complex probably needs to trigger some secondary messengers within the cell. A typical example of how complex the intracellular events may be is illustrated by the outline of the β_2-adrenoreceptor in Box 6.1. If we by effect mean the degree of muscle relaxation, it is not clear why the simple receptor model discussed above should apply.

In order to get a bit more insight into Nature's design of the β_2-receptor, let us analyze it one step further. We see in Box 6.1 that its first action is to activate a certain type of protein, the G protein. The G protein is an example of a so-called transducer protein, and we want to investigate the implications of this stage – why did Nature invent this step?

Let us assume that our drug-receptor complex activates a transducer protein, with the same kind of simple dynamics as above:

$$T + DR \underset{k_{off}}{\overset{k_{on}}{\rightleftharpoons}} T^*,$$

where T^* stands for activated transducer (i.e., the T-DR complex). From this we deduce the differential equation

$$[T^*]' = k_{on}[T][DR] - k_{off}[T^*],$$

with the constraint that $[T^*] + [T] = T_{tot}$. If we find the system in equilibrium then

$$[T^*] = \frac{T_{tot}[DR]}{K_T + [DR]}, \qquad K_T = k_{off}/k_{on}.$$

In order to get this as a function of drug concentration, we insert the expression in equation 6.2 for $[DR]$ to get

$$[T^*] = \frac{T_{tot}R_0 C}{K_T(K_d + C) + R_0 C} = \frac{T_{max}C_u}{K_T' + C},$$

where

$$T_{max} = \frac{T_{tot}R_0}{K_T + R_0}, \quad \text{and} \quad K_T' = \frac{K_T K_d}{K_T + R_0},$$

and C is the unbound drug concentration.

Now assume that there are many receptors for each transducer protein - a situation called the "spare receptor model". This means that $R_0 \gg K_T$, and we have that

$$[T^*] = \frac{T_{tot}C}{K_T' + C}, \quad K_T' = \frac{K_T K_d}{R_0} \ll K_d.$$

If the pharmacological effect is proportional to $[T^*]$, this means that EC_{50} is much smaller than it would have been without the transducer. In other words, Nature has increased the sensitivity of the system by coupling the receptor and the transducer. Note that Nature can play with the sensitivity by increasing (which is called up-regulating the receptor) or decreasing (called down-regulating the receptor) the total amount R_0 of receptors within the cell membrane. Receptors are proteins synthesized by the cell and the amount of them in the cell membrane is the effect of a production/break-down equilibrium.

However, as exemplified by the description in Box 6.1, the intracellular events are typically much more complicated than this model describes and there is often no reason to believe there is a simple functional relationship between the concentration of activated transducer and the effect we measure.

For that reason we may need to take a more empirical approach to the analysis of concentration-effect relationships. If the concentration of drug is C and the effect we measure $E = \Phi(C)$ is a function of it, the assumptions on this function typically include

- $\Phi(0) = 0$,

- there is a maximal effect E_{max} attainable and the effect is monotonously increasing with C (so that $E_{max} = \lim_{C \to \infty} \Phi(C)$).

- the general shape of $\Phi(C)$ is sigmoidal in the sense that there is virtually no effect for small concentrations, then there is a region in which relatively small changes in concentration induce substantial changes in effect leading up to the maximal effect. Further increases in C has then little effect on $\Phi(C)$.

A very useful functional representation of such a function is

$$\Phi(C) = \frac{E_{max} C^\gamma}{EC_{50}^\gamma + C^\gamma},$$

where the parameter γ, which defines the slope of this function, is often called Hill's coefficient. The number EC_{50} is still the concentration that causes half the maximal effect, $E_{max}/2$. This model is usually called the Emax model.

The general shape of such a function is shown in Figure 6.1, where a key feature of the function also is illustrated, namely that it is well approximated by a simple linear function of log-concentration

$$\Phi(C) \approx a + b \ln C,$$

for most of its effect range. The rule of thumb is that this is a valid approximation between 20% and 80% of the effect range. This is useful if our data do not allow us to identify E_{max}.

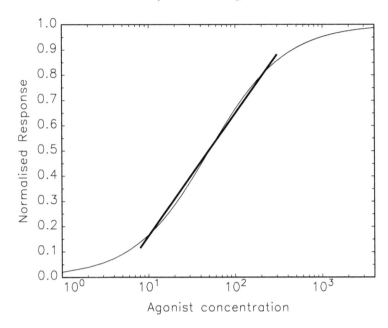

FIGURE 6.1: Illustration of the Emax-function

6.3 Modelling an antagonist

In the previous section we made a simplifying assumption. We assumed that there was an endogenous substance meant by Nature for the receptor. Then we have designed another drug that binds to the same receptor with similar effect. In the analysis we ignored the endogenous substance and only modelled our drug and its relation to the receptor. In real life one could expect a competition for receptor sites for our drug and that of Nature.

We will now remedy the short-coming of the modelling by looking more closely at the interaction between the two substances in their competition for receptor sites. This discussion will allow our drug to have different efficacy when forming a drug-receptor complex, even to the extreme that it has no effect at all. That is the situation we have when our designed drug is a *competitive antagonist*. If the effect is less than that of the endogenous substance, but still positive, we talk about a *partial agonist*.

So let us assume we have two substances, D and A, which both form complexes with the receptor R in the simple way previously discussed, which can be described by the pair of differential equations

$$[DR]' = k_1[D][R] - k_{-1}[DR], \qquad [AR]' = k_2[A][R] - k_{-2}[AR].$$

Here we have that $[R] + [DR] + [AR] = R_0$, which is the constraint that links the two equations. Assume also that the reactions are so fast that they can be assumed to be at equilibrium. We then get a linear system in the pair of concentrations of drug-complexes ($[DR], [AR]$):

$$[D](R_0 - [DR] - [AR]) - K_1[DR] = 0,$$
$$[A](R_0 - [DR] - [AR]) - K_2[AR] = 0,$$

where $K_i = k_{-i}/k_i, i = 1, 2$. Solving for $[DR]$ from the first:

$$[DR] = \frac{[D](R_0 - [AR])}{K_1 + [D]}$$

and inserting into the second gives us

$$[AR] = \frac{R_0[A]}{K_2(1 + [D]/K_1) + [A]}, \qquad [DR] = \frac{R_0[D]}{K_1(1 + [A]/K_2) + [D]}. \qquad (6.4)$$

If we assume that there is no effect whatsoever of the complex $[AR]$, we can compare the expression for $[DR]$ with that of equation 6.3. What we see is that the effect of the antagonist is to modify EC_{50} according to

$$EC_{50}(A) = EC_{50}(0)(1 + [A]/K_2), \qquad (6.5)$$

which corresponds to a shift of the response curve to the right. In other words, the sensitivity to the agonist decreases.

We can rewrite Equation 6.5 as

$$\log(\frac{EC_{50}(A)}{EC_{50}(0)} - 1) = \log[A] - \log K_2,$$

from which we see that if we plot the left hand side versus $\log[A]$ we should get a straight line with slope one. Such a plot is called a *Schild plot*, if we use the base 10 logarithm. The particular concentration for which

$$EC_{50}(A) = 2EC_{50}(0)$$

is denoted A_2, and its negative logarithm (to base 10) pA_2. This number is obtained from the Schild plot as the intersection of the line with the x-axis.

For a partial agonist a simple model is to assume that the effect is proportional to $[DR] + \alpha[AR]$ for some number α in the range (0,1). An antagonist corresponds to the case $\alpha = 0$, and a full agonist to $\alpha = 1$. A short computation shows that

$$[DR] + \alpha[AR] = R_0 \frac{[D]/K_1 + \alpha[A]/K_2}{1 + [A]/K_2 + [D]/K_1} =$$

$$\frac{\alpha R_0[A]}{K_2 + [A]} + \frac{R_0(K_2 + (1 - \alpha)[A])}{K_2 + [A]} \frac{[D]}{K_1(1 + [A]/K_2) + [D]}.$$

To see what this means, assume that we have a background treatment with concentration $[A]$ of the partial antagonist. Then we want to see the concentration response relationship for the full agonist D. This then takes the form

$$E(C) = E_0(A) + (E_{max} - E_0(A))\frac{C}{EC_{50}(1 + [A]/K_2) + C},$$

where $C = [D]$ is the concentration of the agonist and E_{max} and EC_{50} are numbers relating to the agonist itself. So we start at a level defined by the concentration of the partial agonist, after which an increase in the agonist concentration makes us approach the maximal attainable effect. However, the sensitivity to the agonist has decreased! All this is illustrated in Figure 6.2 which shows how the response curve for the agonist looks at different background concentrations of the antagonist. For this example, α was set to 0.7, and the highest concentration of the antagonist is so large that this actually is the baseline response.

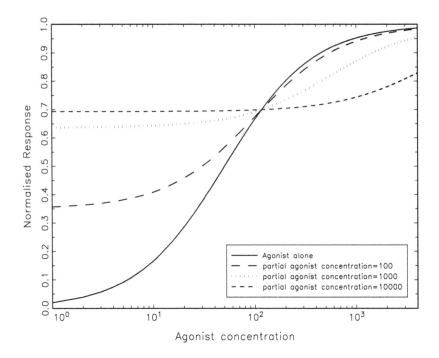

FIGURE 6.2: Illustration on how a background treatment with a partial agonist affects the dose response curve of an agonist

The horizonal shift is, as above, given by the concentration of the partial agonist. The larger the concentration of the partial agonist, the larger will be the baseline effect level, E_0, and the larger will be the horizontal shift. The decreased sensitivity means that treatment with a partial agonist may reduce the ability to respond to an acute need of more agonist.

Since the intracellular events and their connection to the effect measured may be much more complicated, the introduction of Hill's constant in the function $E(C)$ may be necessary. Using formulas derived above, we may then derive at an empirical model that allows us to describe the interaction between the agonist and the antagonist.

Finally, there are also *noncompetitive antagonists* that bind irreversibly to the receptors. The effect of such antagonists is that they reduce the number of available receptors, R_0, by binding to them, which means that they reduce the efficacy of the drug, not the potency, as competitive antagonists do.

6.4   Hysteresis and approaches to PD/PK modelling

The model discussed so far assumes a direct concentration-effect relationship. In fact, the assumption of the previous two sections was that we held the concentrations fixed and measured the effect in equilibrium as a function of these concentrations. This is a situation that can be set up in the laboratory in various *in vitro* experiments. One such experiment, that involves a β_2-agonist, is to take an isolated guinea pig trachea and put it into a dissection bath to which we add drug of different concentrations. The muscular tonus in the trachea can then be measured.

When working *in vivo* we seldom hold the concentration fixed (though it can be done, using a constant infusion). Instead we generally have a time-varying drug concentration and we have effects that vary with time. Even if we plot effect versus concentration, we may, however, not see patterns that resemble a direct concentration-effect of the kind previously discussed.

Figure 6.3 illustrates what we may find. Even though these are artificial data, we can assume that the drug in question is a β_2-agonist, and that the response is a lung function index such that an increase means better lung function. However, the drug should be given orally (could be theophylline), since we want to discuss PD as predicted from PK, and for an inhaled drug we expect effects before we see drug in plasma. We see that the effect has a baseline value E_0 of about 1.9. When giving drug there is an effect in lung function, which is sustained for some time also after the drug has essentially disappeared from plasma. This is made more clear in a graph where we plot effect data versus plasma concentration which is done in the smaller graph in Figure 6.3. Arrows indicate orientation. If we had a direct concentration-effect relationship, we would find a pure graph $E = E(C)$ of a function here.

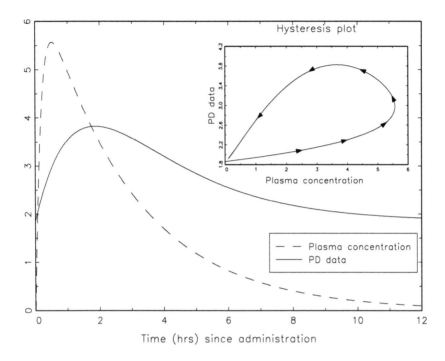

FIGURE 6.3: (Artificial) PK/PD data illustrating hysteresis

The fact that we do not is a property called hysteresis. The word refers to the history dependence of the system.

The purpose of PK/PD modelling is to be able to predict effect from plasma concentrations. If we can do that, we can look for the optimal formulation and dosage regimen of the drug which gives the best absorption profile so that we find the effect profile we want. To achieve this, we need to find a method or model that can account for the hysteresis and from which we can deduce a model that predicts PD from PK.

The natural approach would be to use the differential equation 6.1. Assume a relation between effect and drug-receptor concentration like

$$E = E_{max} f([DR]/R_0)$$

(we normalize so that $E_0 = 0$) for some function $f(u)$ mapping the interval $[0, 1]$ to itself. For example, the simplest assumption, $f(u) = u$, gives us the differential equation

$$E'(t) = k_1 E_{max} C(t) - (k_{-1} + k_1 C(t)) E(t). \tag{6.6}$$

With no drug, this equation becomes

$$E'(t) = -k_{-1} E(t),$$

which means that $E(t) = E(0)e^{-k_{-1}t}$. So, with a half-life time of $\ln(2)/k_{-1}$ the effect returns to the baseline level when drug has disappeared. However, more complicated functions $f(u)$ are not unlikely, accounting for, e.g., intracellular messengers, and this kind of approach to the problem of PK/PD modelling can become very complicated.

Instead we will discuss two modelling approaches that are more generic, and applied with no or only minor biological assumptions, respectively. Both can serve the ultimate purpose of producing predictions of effect from drug concentrations.

The first is the biophase method. The assumption here is that it is not the concentration in the blood that directly determines the effect. For example, bronchial relaxation should be determined by the drug concentrations in the smooth muscles of the bronchi, which is a tissue concentration. But from the discussion in Chapter 4 such a tissue concentration is determined from plasma concentration from a formula like

$$C_T(t) = (H * C)(t).$$

In the well-mixed model, which is the first approximation, we have that $H(t)$ is a mono-exponential function of the form $H(t) = \gamma e^{-\gamma t}$. If we can find a function such that, when plotting the effect E versus C_T the hysteresis has more or less disappeared, we have found a direct concentration effect relationship $E = E(C_T) = E(H * C)$. We need not think of $H * C$ as a true concentration in some tissue, it may be a metabolite or something else. We therefore call this entity the *biophase*, the phase of the drug that has a direct concentration-effect relation, and we do not need to identify it. Its only purpose is to allow PK/PD predictions.

For the data in Figure 6.3 we take $H(t) = \chi e^{-\chi t}, \chi = 0.019$ and then plot the PD effect versus the biophase. This is shown in Figure 6.4 where we see an approximative Emax-relation (the dashed line) between the effect and the biophase. It is not necessarily a good approximation, but it means that we have an approximative PK/PD model.

The other approach we will discuss is a modelling approach that uses some elementary biological assumptions of the process. This type of model is called a *turnover model*. Its basic assumption is that the effect we measure, $E(t)$, in itself is governed by a simple differential equation

$$E'(t) = k_{in} - k_{out}E(t). \tag{6.7}$$

The immediate example would be that $E(t)$ represents the concentration of a substance which is constantly produced with rate k_{in} but eliminated by a first order process. In our guiding example we measure lung function, but we may consider that proportional to the intracellular amount of Ca^{2+} in stores. That is the dynamics of this that is described by Equation 6.7; see Box 6.1.

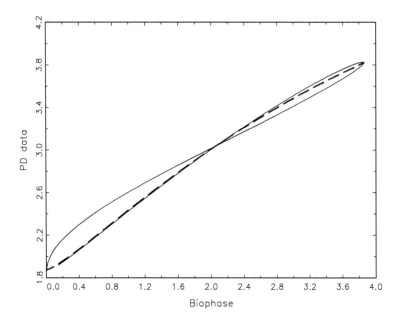

FIGURE 6.4: Hysteresis plot of effect versus biophase with a simple exponential link function between biophase and plasma concentration

The key result of Equation 6.7 is that in equilibrium we have an effect level given by

$$E_0 = \frac{k_{in}}{k_{out}},$$

and the equation governs how we return to this if the system is disturbed.

In our guiding example the drug we give has as its effect to increase the intracellular Ca^{2+} stores. We can model that by letting k_{in} depend on the concentration of drug, for instance, by replacing k_{in} with

$$k_{in}(1 + \frac{E_{max}C}{EC_{50} + C}). \tag{6.8}$$

If the concentration is held constant, this elevates the base level E_0. In fact, in that case it is as model identical with the agonist model in Section 6.2. However, allowing for variable $C(t)$ and inserting that into equation 6.7, where now k_{in} is a function of time, we get a model for which history matters and which exhibits hysteresis. We can estimate constants so that this model fits the original PD-curve as well as possible.

Figure 6.5 shows how well we can describe the true PD data using the two empirical models we have discussed: the biophase model and the turnover model. The coefficients in both models were obtained by a non-linear regression fit to data. We see a close fit to the original data for both methods.

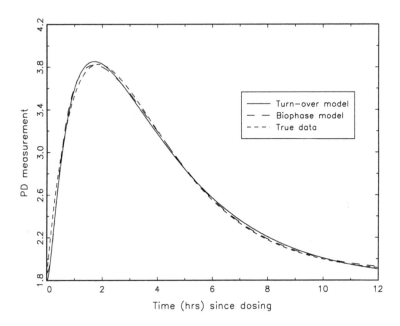

FIGURE 6.5: Illustration on how well the biophase and turnover empirical
models fit to data

Now to predictions. Assume that we can change the formulation of the
drug so that there is a slow release to plasma instead, and that we give three
successive doses with 12 hours interval, with the same dose as we gave in the
original experiment. What will our models predict the effect of lung function
will be? Based on the equations described for the models we can compute
these predictions, which are shown in Figure 6.6.

The interesting point to note from Figure 6.6 is that despite the very close
agreement in Figure 6.5 of the predictions of the two models, there is some
discrepancy in the predictions of the two models for the new situation. The
lesson is that it is not enough to get a close fit (in Figure 6.5) in order to have
found the correct or, rather, a useful model. Instead we need to put the model
to independent tests, where we can compare predictions to experimental data
obtained. This is discussed further in Section 6.6.

6.5   Four types of turn-over models

We will now discuss the turn-over model in some more detail. One of the
nice features of it is that, although it is a considerable simplification of reality,

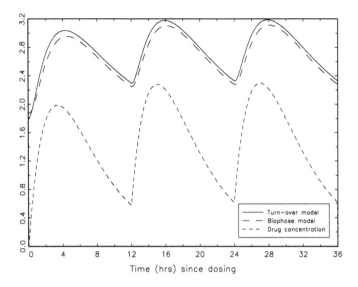

FIGURE 6.6: Predicting effect with a changed formulation

it allows us to at least capture some aspects of what we think the drug does with respect to the effect measured. The logic is based on the differential equation

$$E'(t) = k_{in}(t) - k_{out}E(t), \qquad (6.9)$$

describing drug-free physiology. The reason that we let the production term, k_{in}, depend on time is to allow for a situation that is common in physiology, namely that there is a diurnal variation in what we measure. There are many instances when this is a reasonable first approximation.

Example 6.1

The glucocorticosteroids budesonide and fluticasone that were discussed in Chapter 3 are man-made analogues of an endogenous corticosteroid, namely cortisol. Cortisol is a stress hormone that primarily affects the metabolism of proteins, carbohydrates, and lipids. In addition to this, it has anti-inflammatory and immunosuppressive effects, as well as other effects. It was in order to increase the anti-inflammatory effect that synthetic corticosteroids were made. Cortisol is synthesized by the body in the cortex of the adrenal glands (thus the name corticosteroid), but the regulation of this is a complicated process, involving the so-called hypothalamus-pituitary-adrenal axis (HPA-axis). In plasma, cortisol is bound to more than 90% to a special transport protein, transcortin. It is mainly metabolized in the liver, though a fraction is excreted in the urine. Its half-life is usually given to be between 1 and 1.5 hours.

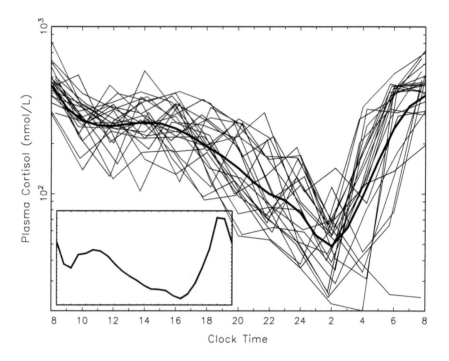

FIGURE 6.7: Cortisol levels over 24 hours

Typical plasma cortisol levels and variability are illustrated in Figure 6.7, which contains cortisol data over a 24 hour period from the study discussed in Section 3.6. These data were obtained on drug free day, showing the pronounced diurnal variation that cortisol levels in plasma exhibit, being at their lowest in the late evening and around midnight and peaking in the early morning.

To apply the turnover model to this, let $E(t) = C(t)$. Assuming that equation 6.9 holds, we can estimate the production rate $k_{in}(t)$ by first numerically differentiating $C(t)$ and then using that, by assumption,

$$k_{in}(t) = C'(t) + k_{el}C(t).$$

We see that the individual plasma cortisol curves in Figure 6.7 are rather "jumpy" in nature. This is believed to be due to short random bursts of cortisol production as response to some internal body stimuli. To model individual curves would therefore be quite challenging and instead we look closer at the (geometric) mean curve, which is displayed as the thick curve embedded among the individual curves in Figure 6.7. The small insert picture in Figure 6.7 shows the deduced production rate for this $(k_{in}(t))$, in which we have assumed a terminal half-life of 1.25 hours.

From the production rate curve we see a diurnal pattern with an increase during early morning, a sharp dip around wake-up time, and then another, somewhat smaller, increase before lunch.

▯

We can express the solution of Equation 6.9 as a convolution equation

$$E(t) = E(0)e^{-k_{out}t} + \int_0^t e^{-k_{out}(t-s)} k_{in}(s) \, ds. \qquad (6.10)$$

As indicated in the previous section, we can now construct a set of four generic PK/PD models of the turnover class. A review of applications for this can be found in [1], from where the examples below are taken. The first type of model in this class was encountered above, in which we replaced $k_{in}(t)$ by the expression in Equation 6.8. We may or may not want to involve a Hill's constant here. If we denote by $E_0(t)$ the baseline solution given by Equation 6.10, and by $E(t)$ the corresponding solution with the input rate given by Equation 6.8, we see that

$$E(t) = E_0(t) + \int_0^t e^{-k_{out}(t-s)} k_{in}(s) \frac{E_{max}C(s)}{EC_{50} + C(s)} \, ds. \qquad (6.11)$$

This situation was considered relevant for the β_2-agonists when we measure lung function.

Another model choice would be relevant for the effect of the steroids budesonide and fluticasone on cortisol. The effect here is a suppression of the production of cortisol, which in its simplest form would correspond to replacing the baseline production rate $k_{in}(t)$ with

$$k_{in}(t)(1 - \frac{C(t)}{IC_{50} + C(t)}). \qquad (6.12)$$

The constant IC_{50} would then represent the concentration that provides us with a 50% inhibition of the production rate. For this model we have the solution

$$E(t) = E_0(t) - \int_0^t e^{-k_{out}(t-s)} k_{in}(s) \frac{C(s)}{IC_{50} + C(s)} \, ds. \qquad (6.13)$$

Again we may or may not want to involve a Hill's constant here.

Example 6.2

Applying the model given by equation 6.13, but including a Hill's constant, to the cortisol data that was measured on the single day administrations of budesonide and fluticasone we get the result shown in Figure 6.8.

In Figure 6.8 we have used the geometric mean plasma concentration curves when fitting the model. The parameter estimates are that the IC_{50} is estimated to 0.41 for budesonide and to 0.21 for fluticasone. This is a ratio of 2,

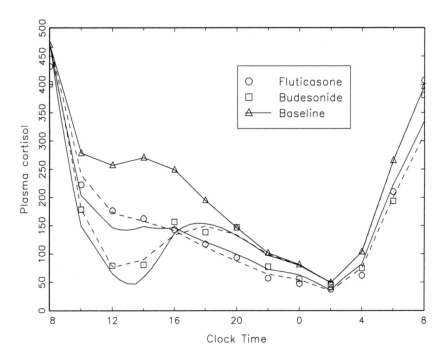

FIGURE 6.8: Geometric mean cortisol levels after a single dose of a steroid treatment. Both data and model predictions (solid lines) are shown.

which may reflect the *in vitro* data claims that fluticasone is twice as potent as budesonide. The estimate of the Hill's coefficient is 6.17 for budesonide and 1.06 for fluticasone. This large difference is needed in order to fit the qualitatively different cortisol curves, with a sharp trough for budesonide and a recoil in late afternoon, but a steady decrease for fluticasone until the early morning burst. The dashed curves in Figure 6.8 will be discussed in Section 6.6.

However, the credibility of this model disappears when one compares the prediction of what should happen after multiple dosing of the steroid treatments with what was actually obtained. These data are not shown. ⬚

For other drugs it is the "degradation rate" that is acted on. If we first assume that it is enhanced by the drug it gives us the differential equation

$$E'(t) = k_{in}(t) - k_{out}(1 + \frac{E_{max}C(t)}{EC_{50} + C(t)})E(t).$$

We can rewrite this differential equation as the integral equation

$$E(t) = E_0(t) - k_{out}E_{max}\int_0^t e^{-k_{out}(t-s)}\frac{C(s)}{EC_{50} + C(s)}E(s)\,ds. \qquad (6.14)$$

The β_2-agonists discussed above provide examples also of this, because they lower the plasma levels of potassium as a systemic side-effect. They stimulate the formation of cAMP (see Box 6.1) which also means that a sodium-potassium pump in the cell membranes is activated. This pumps sodium ions out of the cells and exchanges that for potassium ions, which therefore means a re-distribution of potassium from plasma to the interior of the cells. The model assumes that there is a constant rate of flux of potassium out from cells, k_{in}, into plasma, and that the rate of transport into cells from plasma is a first order process with rate constant k_{out}. It is k_{out} that is regulated by the β_2-agonist. The response $E(t)$ is the plasma concentration of potassium.

The fourth model, with inhibition on the "degradation rate":

$$E'(t) = k_{in}(t) - k_{out}\left(1 - \frac{C(t)}{IC_{50} + C(t)}\right)E(t),$$

gives us another integral equation

$$E(t) = E_0(t) + k_{out}\int_0^t e^{-k_{out}(t-s)}\frac{C(s)}{IC_{50} + C(s)}E(s)\,ds. \qquad (6.15)$$

An example where this has been applied is to the diuretic drug furosemide. It inhibits the reabsorption of Na^+ and Cl^- in parts of the nephron, the ascending part of the loop of Henle, which leads to a decrease in the osmotic pressure that is responsible for water reabsorption from the collecting duct. Its action is therefore to increase the urine flow, which in turn is determined by the glomerular filtration rate, GFR, minus the rate of water reabsorption from tubules and collecting ducts in the kidneys. Furosemide inhibits the reabsorption of water from the collecting ducts of the kidneys, so the model takes $E(t)$ to be the urine volume with $k_{in} = $ GFR.

The convolution formulas 6.13 and 6.11 are convenient in estimation problems, since they replace the problem of solving a non-linear ordinary differential equation with integral estimation for the two first models. Formulas 6.14 and 6.15 can similarly be used, if they first are solved by recursively estimating a sequence $E_n(t)$ of functions, with $E_n(t)$ defined from the integral equation but with $E(t)$ replaced by $E_{n-1}(t)$ on the right hand side. We can start with $E_1(t) = 0$.

We end this section by noting that also the drug-receptor equation 6.6 fits into the general context of a turnover model, since it can be written

$$E'(t) = k_{in}(t) - k_{out}(t)E(t),$$

with

$$k_{in}(t) = k_1 E_{max}C(t), \qquad k_{out}(t) = k_{-1} + k_1 C(t).$$

6.6 Chapter epilogue: Modelling considerations

We end this chapter and this book by a few remarks on modelling in general and PK/PD modelling in particular.

Building models is to a large extent what science is all about. Modelling means making a number of simplifying assumptions and joining them together into an image of reality. The perspective and resolution of that image is defined by the objective of the task. We build models because it gives us a perception of understanding the real world, but the ultimate purpose of any model building is to use it to make some kind of prediction. In some sciences the models are predominantly mathematical; in others they are not. We build models that account for historic development based on, e.g., economic forces or geography, models that are expressed in words only. Models in medicine are mostly also expressed free of mathematical formulae (or only very simple ones). In physics it is the opposite – models are almost always expressed in mathematical equations.

Sometimes we model without noting it. Even the simple concept of a plasma concentration is a model. It is something that is measured in the test tube after having mixed plasma obtained from a particular vein for a short period of time. It is a kind of mean value of a true concentration, which varies both with time and position within the blood vessel. It is a quantitative measure which defines a model concept, the concentration in plasma.

Building a model means identifying a limited number of building blocks and relationships between them. In doing this we make various simplifications of a complex reality and, by definition, any model therefore represents only an approximation of the real system. When modelling we first need to identify the objective of the exercise, and then to make the appropriate simplifying hypothesis to allow the construction of a model that both is simple enough to be understood but also a sufficiently good representation of the relevant parts of the reality so that the objective can be achieved. The validity of the model can only be assessed in the context of the purpose for which it was built.

Mathematical modelling does not differ in essence from any other kind of modelling. The difference between a mathematical and a non-mathematical model is only that a special language, mathematics, is used to express the model. This typically increases precision in the model description, since mathematical formulae require clarity in concepts and the relations connecting these concepts.

A mathematical model consists of a number of quantitative measures together with a set of equations connecting these measures to a degree adequate for the purposes for which the model has been constructed. For PK/PD models these equations are typically differential equations or differential-integral equations. In this context one distinguishes between empirical and theoretical models. These are two extremes of how model building can be approached. An empirical model is a description that is driven by the data we have, whereas a theoretical model is derived from theoretical understanding of the system under study. For example, the perfusion limited physiological model studied in Section 4.4.2 can be considered to be a theoretical model since it starts from our knowledge of the human body, whereas the modelling of a drug discussed in Chapter 5 to a large extent is an empirical modelling approach. A theoretical model may be very complex, and a simplification of the model may be needed. How this is done depends on the purpose of the modelling, but an illustration is the approximation of the theoretical physiological model in Section 4.4.2 by a mamillary three-compartment model that was done in Section 5.3. This involves lumping together certain organs and thereby reducing a ten-compartment model to a three-compartment model.

Almost all models are neither purely empirical, nor purely theoretical. The standard PK model discussed in Chapter 2 is to a large extent empirical, but not purely so. In fact, the basic relation between volume $V(t)$ and clearance $CL(t)$ after a bolus dose D is governed by the equation

$$(V(t)C(t))' = -CL(t)C(t), \quad C(0) = D/V(0).$$

From a modelling perspective we can assume that $V(t) = V$ is constant, and let the resulting function $CL(t)$ describe the full dynamics. However, that does not conform with the theoretical knowledge about drug elimination from the body we have. So instead we insert such knowledge by pre-specifying a shape for $CL(t)$, e.g., a constant, and then deduce $V(t)$. In this way the model is a mixture between a theoretical and an empirical model.

The equations in a mathematical PK/PD model typically have a number of unknown coefficients, parameters in the model which we may need to estimate from data. That we have a good fit to the data after this fitting procedure does not guarantee that we have found an appropriate model. There are many models that can be fitted to a given, often limited, set of PK/PD data. That a good fit to data does not guarantee that a model is correct is illustrated by the discussion of PK/PD models for the β_2-agonist, relating lung function and plasma concentrations, which was made above. We fitted two different models to the data and both model fits were very accurate. But they are based on different assumptions. And neither of these is true. In fact, for that example there is no true PK/PD model, since what was done was that we took two functions,

$$C(t) = 1.07(e^{-0.006t} - e^{-0.096t}), \quad E(t) = 1.86 + 5(e^{-0.008t} - e^{-0.01t}),$$

and made the analysis on them, with no assumption of a cause-effect relationship. But obviously there is a relationship between them, since time connects them, and that is what is displayed in the hysteresis plot.

More model parameters to estimate typically give you more possibilities to obtain a good fit, compared to fewer parameters. Consider the steroid suppression data of Example 6.2. An alternative model to the one analyzed there would be a biophase model looking something like

$$E(t) = E_0(t)\Phi((H * C)(t)),$$

where $\Phi(u)$ is an Emax-model and $H(t)$ a monoexponential biophase transfer function acting on the concentration $C(t)$ of the administered steroid. If we fit that model to data, we actually get a better fit, as shown by the dashed curves in Figure 6.8, than the one obtained with the turn-over model. However, this model contains one more parameter per steroid: the number of parameters in the turn-over model is the same as the number of parameters in the Emax-model (remember that we took k_{out} as given in the turn-over model for cortisol in order to be able to deduce $k_{in}(t)$ for the base case), and there is one extra parameter defining $H(t)$.

We do however not like this biophase model for the cortisol data, since it is hard to reconcile with what we believe we know about cortisol dynamics in the body. We believe that the exogenously administered steroids act via inhibiting the production of cortisol. In model building in biology, it is probably a very good idea to require that the model should make sense. That a model should make sense is not a universal requirement when modelling. Quantum physics is a field one is warned against trying to "understand" – it is more of a formalistic machine that provides you with very accurate predictions. But it gives no unique interpretation of what is going on. Biology at the present stage should probably be considered to be different from quantum physics. Modelling in biology is in its infancy and we should always be able to make some sense out the model.

So, for biological reasons, we prefer the turn-over model of Example 6.2 over the biophase approach, despite the poorer fit. But we see a need to improve upon the turn-over model and replace it with something that makes biological sense but provides a better fit to data. How can this be done? Two immediate suggestions are:

1. The exogenously administered steroids had some clear distribution phases. Should not cortisol exhibit that as well? This means that we modify the equation for $E(t)$ to

$$E'(t) = k_{in}(t) + (h * E)(t) - \kappa E(t)$$

for some function $h(t)$ and constant κ.

2. The regulation of cortisol production is more complicated than what the present model accounts for. Cortisol production in the adrenal gland is triggered by a hormone, ACTH, produced by the pituitary gland. Production of this in turn is regulated by a hormone from the hypothalamus. This means that there are plenty of opportunities to model the production function $k_{in}(t)$. Under baseline conditions this could, e.g., be some

highly non-linear function of cortisol concentration which is such that production is initiated when levels go below a certain threshold.

We do not pursue any of these ideas since it would lead us into modelling a type of physiological dynamics that is outside the scope of this book.

The ultimate purpose of any model is to make predictions, to use the model to predict what will happen in a new set of circumstances and compare that prediction with the true outcome, that is, if possible. We may not want to, or many not be able to, test the predictions, like in war games or greenhouse effects, but we need to check the validity of our model in some way. For example, in Example 6.2, the model makes a claim about how plasma concentrations of an exogenous steroid affect cortisol concentrations, and if the model is valid, it should apply also to the steady state situation. We have data for that, which are data independent of the data that we actually fitted the model parameters on, so we can use that for validation. If the model reproduces the observed data, we have found support for our model.

But support is not a final proof of the model. In fact, there is no such thing as a true model. "All models are wrong, but some are useful" as the saying is. By definition a model is always wrong since it involves a simplification of reality. If it does not involve a simplification, it is not a model but a description of reality. How complex a model should be depends on what it is to be used for. In fact, we still compute spacecraft trajectories using Newton's mechanics ignoring both general relativity and quantum effects. We use a model we know is wrong in the sense that it does not account for everything we know, but which gives good enough predictions for the problem at hand. Similarly, in PK/PD modelling, it is the purpose of the modelling that defines how complex the model needs to be.

With these remarks our tour of the theory of pharmacokinetics comes to a conclusion. Hopefully the presentation has given the reader a better understanding of PK modelling. The ideas discussed here can of course also be applied, in suitably modified form, in related areas, like the analysis of metabolic and endocrinologic systems.

Appendix A

Linear ordinary differential equations

A.1 Linear differential equations

A univariate ordinary differential equation is one in which we, for given functions $a(t), f(t)$, try to find a function $x(t)$ such that

$$x'(t) + a(t)x(t) = f(t), \tag{A.1}$$

and for which we assume a start condition $x(0) = x_0$. To solve such an equation, we define a function $A(t)$ such that $A'(t) = a(t)$ and $A(0) = 0$, and multiply equation A.1 by $e^{A(t)}$. Using the product formula for differentiation we can then rewrite the equation as

$$(e^{A(t)}x(t))' = e^{A(t)}f(t).$$

Integrating this relation from 0 to t shows that

$$e^{A(t)}x(t) = x(0) + \int_0^t e^{A(s)}f(s)\,ds$$

from which we deduce that

$$x(t) = U(t,0)x_0 + \int_0^t U(t,s)f(s)\,ds, \tag{A.2}$$

where

$$U(t,s) = e^{A(s)-A(t)}.$$

The function $x(t) = U(t,s), t > s$, for fixed s solves the problem

$$x'(t) + a(t)x(t) = 0, \quad x(s) = 1. \tag{A.3}$$

This can be generalized to higher dimensions, where $a(t)$ is a $p \times p$-matrix, insofar as we define a function $U(t,s)$ from a matrix generalization of equation A.3,

$$U'(t,s) + a(t)U(t,s) = 0, \quad U(s,s) = I,$$

where I is the $p \times p$-identity matrix. (Differentiation is with respect to t.) Then the integral equation in equation A.2 holds true.

The most important case to us is the case when $a(t)$ is a constant matrix, so that $A(t) = at$. Then

$$U(t, s) = e^{-a(t-s)}$$

where the right hand side can be defined for square matrices as it is defined in the univariate case, as a convergent power series. However, methods for computing it usually employ diagonalization methods. Assuming a non-degenerate case with distinct eigenvalues, this means that we write the matrix a as $T^{-1}\Lambda T$, where Λ is the diagonal matrix of eigenvalues λ_i, and T a matrix of eigenvectors. Then

$$e^{-at} = \sum_{k=0}^{\infty} \frac{(-T^{-1}\Lambda Tt)^k}{k!} = T^{-1}\left(\sum_{k=0}^{\infty} \frac{-(\Lambda t)^k}{k!}\right)T = T^{-1}e^{-\Lambda t}T,$$

where $e^{-\Lambda t}$ is the diagonal matrix of functions $e^{-\lambda_i t}$. It follows that $e^{-at}x_0$ is a sum of exponentials of the eigenvalues for all initial conditions x_0.

In this case of constant coefficients the integral in equation A.2 becomes a convolution:

$$x(t) = e^{-at}x_0 + (e^{-at} * x)(t).$$

A.2   Explicit formulas for 2-by-2 systems

In this section we will explicitly derive a solution to a homogenous 2-by-2 system of ordinary differential equations

$$x_1'(t) = ax_1(t) + bx_2(t), \quad x_1(0) = x_0$$
$$x_2'(t) = cx_1(t) + dx_2(t), \quad x_2(0) = 0.$$

The solution so obtained is used in the discussion on the two-compartment model in Section 5.2. We will derive the solution using matrix theory, and allow complex numbers in the computations. From above, we then know that the solution of this can be written as the sum of the two exponential functions $e^{\lambda_i t}, i = 1, 2$, where λ_1, λ_2 are eigenvalues to the coefficient matrix

$$A = \begin{pmatrix} a & b \\ c & d \end{pmatrix}.$$

We determine the coefficients as follows: put

$$x_1(t) = B_{11}e^{\lambda_1 t} + B_{12}e^{\lambda_2 t}, \quad x_2(t) = B_{21}e^{\lambda_1 t} + B_{22}e^{\lambda_2 t}.$$

The start condition then gives us the relations

$$B_{11} + B_{12} = x_0, \qquad B_{22} = -B_{21}$$

so that

$$x_1(t) = B_1 e^{\lambda_1 t} + (x_0 - B_1) e^{\lambda_2 t}, \qquad x_2(t) = B_2 (e^{\lambda_1 t} - e^{\lambda_2 t}),$$

where $B_1 = B_{11}$ and $B_2 = B_{22}$.

The eigenvalues in turn are the solution to the quadratic

$$(a - \lambda)(d - \lambda) - bc = 0,$$

and therefore given by

$$\frac{1}{2}\left((a + d) \pm \sqrt{(a - d)^2 + 4bc}\right).$$

Also note that

$$\lambda - a = (d - a \pm \sqrt{(a - d)^2 + 4bc})/2$$

so that

$$(\lambda_1 - a)(\lambda_2 - a) = ((d - a)^2 - ((a - d)^2 + 4bc)/4 = bc.$$

The vector $\begin{pmatrix} B_1 \\ B_2 \end{pmatrix}$ is eigenvector to the eigenvalue λ_1 and $\begin{pmatrix} x_0 - B_1 \\ -B_2 \end{pmatrix}$ is eigenvector to the other eigenvalue λ_2, since they are the coefficients of the corresponding exponentials in the solution. The eigenvector to λ_i is determined from the equations

$$(a - \lambda_i)x_1 + bx_2 = 0, \qquad cx_1 + (d - \lambda_i)x_2 = 0$$

which means that it is $t \begin{pmatrix} b \\ \lambda_i - a \end{pmatrix}$, and we therefore have that

$$B_2/B_1 = (\lambda_1 - a)/b, \qquad (B_1 - x_0)/B_2 = b/(\lambda_2 - a).$$

The first equation here shows that $B_2 = B_1(\lambda_1 - a)/b$ and inserting that into the second one we get

$$B_1 - x_0 = B_1(\lambda_1 - a)/(\lambda_2 - a)$$

which gives us the final solution

$$B_1 = \frac{x_0(\lambda_2 - a)}{\lambda_2 - \lambda_1}, \qquad B_2 = \frac{x_0(\lambda_1 - a)(\lambda_2 - a)}{b(\lambda_2 - \lambda_1)} = \frac{x_0 c}{\lambda_2 - \lambda_1}.$$

Collecting this information we find that

$$x_1(t) = \frac{x_0}{\lambda_2 - \lambda_1}((\lambda_2 - a)e^{\lambda_1 t} - (\lambda_1 - a)e^{\lambda_2 t}), \qquad x_2(t) = \frac{x_0 c}{\lambda_2 - \lambda_1}(e^{\lambda_1 t} - e^{\lambda_2 t}).$$

The eigenvalues are real and of same sign if $bc - ad < 0$ and $(a-d)^2 + 4bc > 0$. The latter is fulfilled if b and c have the same sign. In our case, with

$$a = -(k_{cp} + k_{ce}), \quad b = k_{pc}, \quad c = k_{cp}, \quad d = -(k_{pc} + k_{pe}),$$

these conditions are fulfilled and we see that we get negative eigenvalues. If we therefore substitute λ_i for $-\lambda_i$ and assume that $\lambda_1 > \lambda_2$ we get

$$x_1(t) = \frac{x_0}{\lambda_1 - \lambda_2}\left(-(\lambda_2 + a)e^{-\lambda_1 t} + (\lambda_1 + a)e^{-\lambda_2 t}\right) \tag{A.4}$$

$$x_2(t) = \frac{Db}{\lambda_1 - \lambda_2}\left(e^{-\lambda_2 t} - e^{-\lambda_1 t}\right) \tag{A.5}$$

Introduce the notation $Z = \lambda_1 - \lambda_2 = \sqrt{(a-d)^2 + 4bc}$. We then have the following equations

$$a + d - Z = -2\lambda_1, \quad a + d + Z = -2\lambda_2, \quad x_0(\lambda_1 + a) = B_2 Z,$$

which can be rewritten as

$$Z = \lambda_1 - \lambda_2, \qquad a = B_2 Z / x_0 - \lambda_1, \qquad d = -2\lambda_1 + Z - a.$$

Insert this above and we get

$$Z^2 = (a-d)^2 + 4bc \implies bc = (Z^2 - (a-d)^2)/4.$$

Appendix B

Key notations

The following table lists a few key notations that are uniquely defined in the text. Some notation is context dependent and not listed.

Notation	Meaning
$a(t)$	absorption/input rate function
AUC	Area Under the Curve, PK notation for $I(f)$
AUMC	Area Under the Moment Curve, PK notation for $E(f)$
$C(t)$	Drug concentration in a particular blood compartment
$C_u(t)$	Unbound drug concentration
$CL(t)$	Clearance function, $e(t) = CL(t)C(t)$
CL_{av}	Average clearance, $D/I(C)$
CL_{int}	Intrinsic clearance
D	Dose, amount of drug ever present at the site of observation
E	Extraction ratio over an organ
$E(t)$	The pharmacodynamic response function
$e(t)$	Drug elimination rate function
$E(f)$	The integral $\int_0^\infty t f(t)\,dt$
F	Fraction of dose given that present at the site of observation
f_u	Fraction unbound drug
$h(t)$	Transfer function in peripheral compartment
k_a	Absorption rate, for first order absorption
λ_{el}	Terminal elimination rate
$I(f)$	The integral $\int_0^\infty f(t)\,dt$
$M(t)$	Amount of drug in body at time t
MRT	Mean Residence Time for a drug molecule in blood, $E(e)/I(e)$
MRT_{app}	Apparent Mean Residence Time, defined by $E(C)/I(C)$
MRT_{iv}	Apparent Mean Residence Time of a bolus dose
MTT	Mean Transit Time, of a particular compartment
NCA	Non-Compartmental Analysis
Q	Blood flow
Q_c	Cardiac output
R_{ac}	Accumulation ratio based on AUC
R_{pac}	The predicted accumulation ratio based on AUC from single dose data
$t_{1/2}$	Terminal elimination half-life, $\ln(2)/k_{el}$

Notation	Meaning
t_{circ}	The time it takes a drug molecule to make one circulation in the body
$V(t)$	Distributional volume function, defined by $M(t) = V(t)C(t)$
V_c	Volume of the central compartment
V_d	Terminal distributional volume, CL_{av}/λ_{el}
V_{ss}	Volume in steady state, defined by $CL_{av} \cdot \mathrm{MRT}$

References

[1] William J. Jusko and Hui C. Ko. Physiologic indirect response models characterize diverse types of pharmacodynamic effects. *Clinical Pharmacology and Therapeutics*, 56(4):406–419, October 1994.

[2] Anders Källén and Lars Thorsson. Drug disposition analysis: A comparison between budesonide and fluticasone. *Journal of Pharmacokinetics and Pharmacodynamics*, 30(4):239–256, 2003.

[3] Lars Thorsson, Staffan Edsbäcker, Anders Källén and Claes-Göran Löfdahl. Pharmacokinetics and systemic activity of fluticasone via Diskus®and pMDI, and of budesonide via Turbuhaler®. *Br. J. Clin. Pharmacol.*, 52:529–538, 2001.

[4] Johannes H. Proost. The application of a numerical deconvolution technique in the assessment of bioavailability. *J. Pharm. Sci.*, 74(10):1135–1136, 1985.

[5] Douglas Shepard Riggs. *The Mathematical Approach to Physiological Problems: A Critical Primer*. The M.I.T. Press, first edition, 1970.

[6] Malcolm Rowland and Thomas N. Tozer. *Clinical Pharmacokinetics: Concepts and Appplications*. Lea & Febiger, third edition, 1995.

Index